BOTH SIDES OF SELECTION

Finding and filling jobs in nursing and the health services

MARTIN EDIS

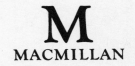

MACMILLAN

© Martin Edis and Nursing Times 1990

First edition 1990

Published by
MACMILLAN EDUCATION LTD
Houndmills, Basingstoke, Hampshire RG21 2XS
and London
Companies and representatives
throughout the world

Typeset by Footnote Graphics,
Warminster, Wiltshire

Printed in Great Britain by
Billing & Sons Ltd, Worcester

British Library Cataloguing in Publication Data
Edis, Martin
Both sides of selection : finding and filling jobs in
nursing and the health services.
1. Great Britain. Health services. Personnel. Recruitment.
I. Title
362.10683
ISBN 0–333–54239–8

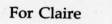

For Claire

CONTENTS

vii

LIST OF FIGURES

PREFACE

This book has been written for all of the parties involved in selection. It is about how to manage the selection process, whether you be a candidate or a selector.

It is written primarily for people in the nursing profession, but its contents are equally applicable to other professionals, particularly those working in the UK National Health Service.

I shall concentrate a great deal on the source of most people's concerns – the interview. I will explain how it can be conducted most effectively, and give advice to candidates on how they can put themselves across confidently.

Nearly everyone has memories of interviews that have been gruelling and frustrating rituals, neither positive nor useful. My objective is to ensure that the interview process will not be an ordeal nor an exercise in miscommunication, but that, at least some of the time, it will become a rewarding and useful experience for all parties.

Generally, I have used the female gender in this book, as doing so is appropriate in the context I am writing about. Readers are, of course, free to substitute 'he' for 'she' where they so desire.

Part One of this book is written for candidates, and Part Two for selectors. However, there is material throughout the book to interest both parties. Readers will also find some similarity between Chapters 1 and 14. This is because the issues covered are relevant to both parties, and the material has been repeated for completeness.

To illustrate many aspects of the selection process, I will be asking you to follow the progress of Sally Robinson, candidate, and Shirley Garnett and Miss Williams, interviewers. Their experiences are described in a narrative called 'The day of judgement'. This appears in instalments at the beginning of Part One and Part Two, and it is concluded at the end of Chapter 25.

ACKNOWLEDGEMENTS

Several of the chapters in this book appeared in their original form in *Nursing Times*. I would like to express my gratitude to several of the original authors for agreeing to let me use and adapt their material in this book.

The authors to whom thanks are due are Jane Schober[1] (for parts of Chapter 2), Ray Rowden[2] (for parts of Chapter 3) and Anne Smith[3] (for much of Chapter 25). Chapters 12 and 23 include original articles by Jill Fardell and Andrew Cole, both of *Nursing Times*, which I have used in their entirety. Jill Fardell commissioned the original series of articles and provided many ideas and much advice on the development of this book. I must give particular thanks to Jill Baker, who contributed Chapter 5 and offered invaluable help with the text.

[1] Jane Schober MN SRN RCNT DipN (Lond) DipNEd RNT is Principal Lecturer (Nursing) at Leicester Polytechnic.

[2] Ray Rowden SRN RMN ONCNC MBIM LHSM is general manager, priority services, West Lambeth Health Authority, and an associate editor of *Nursing Times*.

[3] Anne Smith RGN is assistant general manager (central community services) in the Acute and Community Services Unit, East Surrey Health Authority.

THE CANDIDATE

This book is divided into a candidates' part and an interviewers' part. In this part, we look at the interview from the candidates' point of view. To illustrate many aspects of the selection process, I will be asking you to follow the progress of Sally Robinson, candidate, and Shirley Garnett and Miss Williams, interviewers. Their experiences are described in a narrative called 'The day of judgement'. This appears in instalments before Part One and Part Two, and is concluded at the end of the book.

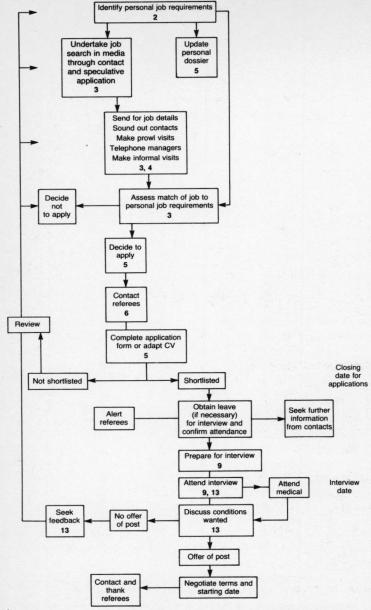

Flowchart A *The selection process for the candidate* (numbers refer to chapters)

THE DAY OF JUDGEMENT – THE INITIATION

On a cold morning in January, Sally set out for her job interview for a senior staff nurse post, grade E.

As she waited anxiously for the bus, a number of things were on her mind. She was concerned that she would get there on time, and not arrive flustered and disorganised. She realised that she should have checked the time of the buses, to find out how long the journey might take at that time in the morning.

When the bus finally arrived, and moved off, she was beginning to panic. Did she leave the job description with the notes of the questions she wanted to ask on her kitchen table? She rummaged in vain through her handbag. It was not there.

Later on, she tried to focus on the interview. What will the panel be like? Will they be friendly, and ask questions she can answer confidently, or will she face trick questions, where she will either make a fool of herself by saying all the wrong things or pass into an embarrassed silence?

As the bus reached her destination she got up, glancing for the umpteenth time at her watch. Is it really that time? If she walked fast down the hill, she would just about make it. She did not want to arrive looking dishevelled. She remembered that interviews always seem to run late – but it would give a bad impression to fail to arrive on time.

She finally entered the unfamiliar building, and went up to the rather stiff-looking lady on the reception desk. Is this the place she will be working in, if she is successful?

The nurse manager who gave her a reference had asked her whether she felt it was really the right job for her. Sally did not want to lose face at that moment by admitting that she was not at all sure. The publicity for the job had made it seem exciting and interesting. Now her managers 'knew she was off' it might discourage them from considering her for the sister's post coming up soon. Perhaps her application had partly been to spite them for not shortlisting her for the previous vacancy?

Sally tried to put these thoughts out of her mind. The lift reached the third floor, the door opened and outside it a lady was waiting. 'Miss Robinson?'

'Yes', said Sally.

'Hello, did you have a good journey? I'm afraid one of the panel is still on her way. Perhaps you'd like a cup of coffee while you are waiting?'

Meanwhile, Shirley Garnett, the person they are waiting for, was stuck in a traffic jam a couple of miles away. After dealing with a few minor crises on the wards that morning, she had rung to say she would be late, grabbed the pile of application forms on her desk and dashed off to her car. Shirley did not really want to have to do interviewing that morning at all. It was not something she enjoyed.

She had to remember the questions she usually asked, and find time to look at the application forms before the candidate came in. She always took them home the previous night and intended to look at them, but never did. Instead, she would rely on her colleague, Miss Williams, who was an old hand.

Fortunately, her colleague, Miss Williams, was always meticulous. She would be aware of everything each candidate had written, and would already have made some firm judgements on the candidate and have a list of questions ready. For her, bad handwriting was an infallible sign of unreliability. Miss Williams did have the reputation of being rather arbitrary in her judgements at times, but no one could accuse her of not being thorough in putting candidates through the mill. She prided herself on not being easily fooled by glib talk, and tended to favour the older, more mature person, especially if they had trained somewhere that she knew.

The interviewers bustled to the room and hustled to their seats. They pulled out Sally's application form and quickly read through it. Miss Williams voiced some misgivings about Sally's experience and about the way she had completed some sections. Shirley Garnett really wanted more time to discuss their strategy as interviewers, but she was a little afraid to reveal to Miss Williams anything that might be taken as a lack of competence. To Miss Williams the purpose would be obvious. Her interviewing would follow a well-tried pattern. As it was just on nine thirty, she decided to call Sally in without further ado.

Sally entered timidly, not at all sure what would happen next. Her mind went blank, and her stomach was turning. She could hardly speak.

'Welcome Miss Robinson. Can you tell us why you have applied for this job?'

*   *   *

4

From these few details, we will not find it difficult to predict what might happen. Sally is probably not going to have an easy time. As she is nervous, and unprepared, she will not give of her best. Faced with one nervous interviewer, and another one possessing certain prejudices who intimidates her, the interview is unlikely to run smoothly. Sally's lack of preparation will probably let her down.

If she is offered the job, she may still have doubts about it, yet not wish to lose face by refusing it. She is unlikely to be in the best position to judge.

If she is not considered suitable, will anyone be any the wiser for the experience? Miss Williams and Shirley Garnett will never in fact know whether their questions reveal the truth, or whether their judgements will turn out to be right or wrong. They do not take on the people they do not like, and the people they think they like are sometimes disappointing.

We shall return to this imaginary situation later, to look more closely at what goes on in selecting people, from both sides of the table.

Chapter 1

PERSPECTIVES ON SELECTION

THE TRADITION OF INTERVIEWING

In all the years that people have been selected for jobs, it is unfortunate in some ways that some method other than the interview has not become popular. Psychologists are always telling us not to rely on the interview for selection – they can prove that interview judgements are often poor. Everyone can do it badly – but this is never brought home to people, except in the case of their disasters.

Everyone wants to do interviews. There is an understandable compulsion to meet the people who will be working with us, and this leads us easily to want to turn this meeting into an assessment procedure. So the meeting becomes a 'conversation with a purpose', and the tradition shows no sign of disappearing.

However, unlike other conversations with a purpose, like a clinical interview, the job interview has become a rather frightening ritual, where neither side is particularly natural, and the candidate often does not do justice to herself. We all know really competent people who come over like idiots at job interviews. We all know very clever people whose interviewing style is hopeless. If the interview is going to persist as a selection device, and it will until something better comes along, everyone must seek to develop the same level of competence that they would expect to have in a clinical or professional role.

THE COMPLIANT NURSE

The traditional culture has been authoritarian and has discouraged individual competition. It is assumed that matron (or ster) knows best. Self-assertion has not been encouraged, and has not been the way to get on. Demonstrable clinical pro-.ciency and reliability have been recognised through personal patronage and recommendation, and this has been the way to get up the nursing ladder. These traditions have made the average nurse reluctant to market herself to employers and to sell herself at the interview.

In the commercial world, the emphasis has been on assertive, competitive self-promotion – even to the extent of overselling oneself – and of hard negotiation about terms being offered. In the world of nursing, on the other hand, the interview has been more like an extension of clinical assessment, and the terms and conditions have definitely not been negotiable. Many nurses have been conditioned to feel inadequate in interviews. For some, the fear of assessment makes them neurotic. The confident, practical nurse who has no fear of clinical horrors that would make a lay person faint, or who confidently undertakes very difficult and complex counselling, is often reduced to a jelly at the thought of having to attend an interview.

For a long time, nurses have tended to undervalue the skills they have – to see themselves as second-class citizens in comparison with other professionals. Some have seen this as a consequence of nursing being a female-dominated profession.

WHY THE MYSTERY?

There has been little advice given to nurses about selection and the job interview. If I can explain it as simply a set of procedures, it may well become less of a mystery. I am sure that nurses, who are trained to deal with the unexpected, who often have superb skills with people, and who are used to being assessed, should not really have difficulties, once they know what the procedure is about.

Many nurse managers have had no proper training, and are nervous, often as much as candidates are. Again, given a knowledge of sound procedure, and a systematic approach, it will be relatively easy for them to use their existing skills to carry out a job interview confidently and well.

THE JOB SEARCH IN THE NINETIES

Whatever has happened in the past, all the trump cards will be held by the candidate from now on. There will be an insatiable demand for qualified people, and particularly for nurses.

Conroy and Stidston's research has indicated that there will be a reduction of 31% in the numbers of school leavers between 1983 and 1993. It is reasonable to assume that the NHS will suffer a proportionately greater reduction than this.

There has been a reduction of almost 30% in the numbers entering nursing training over the period. This allows for the reduction in pupil nurses, but also incorporates a 10% reduction in student nurses. Numbers had even begun to decline in 1982/3, which was the peak year for school leavers.

Another key characteristic of the NHS is its reliance on a very highly qualified workforce – which constitutes only 18% of the labour market. Estimates of the workforce in the Oxford Region alone suggest that one-half would have obtained five 'O' levels and above. The extent to which the NHS can continue with current expectations of attainment is questionable.

Given these factors, and the increasing demand for qualified staff, it has been estimated that one out of every three appropriately qualified females would have to be recruited for the NHS in 1993 – an impossible task. Competition within the 'service sector' will also be increasing.

Recruiting more males, part-time staff and mature entrants might help, but will not provide solutions. Urgent attention will need to be given to retention of staff and to the mix of skills required.

The implications

For the candidate

At first sight, this is good news for candidates – a wider choice of opportunities and very much a 'seller's market' if you are qualified. But think for a moment – might not this in itself raise some problems? There is bound to be some high-powered and persuasive marketing of jobs. Even mediocre ones will be dressed up in all kinds of fancy wrapping. Not only is there likely to be a vast range of vacancies, there may also be a bewildering variety of inducements to fill them. Mature employees and part-timers, including working mothers, will find employers taking their needs much more seriously – the horizons open to them will expand rapidly. Hence the need:

to identify what you want
to make sure you are not being taken for a ride or flattered by the opportunities you will be offered
- to know what you can negotiate for yourself
- to be credible and effective in presenting yourself.

Up until now, many nurses have had attitudes like:

I know I am a good nurse. Why should I have to perform at an interview?

I am fine on the ward, where I know what I am doing. I rarely have interviews; I do not know what to expect or how to behave.

I have given up ideas of pursuing a career while my children need me

Now you will be entering a much more competitive era. You will need to market your talents effectively, if you want to take advantage of the undoubted opportunities.

Given the shortage of skilled labour, you will be able, if you want, to sell the skills you have acquired in nursing to employers outside the health sector. If you look at the summary on page 20 of the skills used by nurses, you will find that they are many and varied, and extremely useful to such employers. Unless you are able to convince an employer that you have these skills, the opportunities will go begging.

On the other hand, as a candidate, your interview skills will provide you with the passport to better things.

For the employer

Undoubtedly, there will be greater competition for scarce, professionally qualified staff. People will start to spend more money, to make jobs more attractive and market them better. Employers will feel the need to offer inducements to attract new staff, and to hang on to existing staff. They will offer better opportunities and conditions, like education.

There will be a need to attract more male staff and more mature staff. Employers will have to go out of their way to make jobs flexible and attractive to part-timers, who will be much in demand everywhere.

They may lower their selection standards – and certainly they will redesign jobs to enable less skilled people to do the work that has to be done. This means, incidentally, that the professional staff will be expected to supervise these less skilled people and to teach them – putting a greater premium on these particular skills.

For the recruitment and selection process

The balance of power will change. This will probably not affect the way many employers do things. Many will still keep candidates waiting, and give them little chance to ask questions. They will not allow candidates to negotiate the conditions of work that are important to them, like flexible hours or access to certain facilities and training.

However, candidates will increasingly be able to pick and choose their employers, and the ones that adapt to this fact, by offering candidates access and choices, will be the winners. One indication of this is likely to be the increasing perception of the selection process as a two-way affair and as an open process.

If professional staff are hard to come by, one strategy might be to dispense with selection altogether. However, if it is going to require such effort and expense to find qualified staff, and to lure them away from other hungry employers, it might seem rather important to pick the right ones – people whose motivation will be right for that particular job, or whose performance will be adequate.

So it would seem that, even if employers are less fussy (that is, have lower selection standards), there will be a need to ensure 'value for money', and that the selection process itself does not turn people away or give them a bad reputation.

Whether as a candidate or as an interviewer, your skills will never be more needed. This book is intended to help you make sure that you are confident and competent in any job interview situation, on either side of the table.

THE KEY PROCESSES

The book is divided into a 'candidates' part' and an 'interviewers' part'. Yet, in fact, many of the same processes and skills are involved in making the interaction one where the needs of both parties are likely to be met. For both parties, success is about finding the right match. Several processes are involved.

Investigation

Both parties will need to do some preliminary investigation in some depth, to be sure they know what they each want. As a

11

candidate, this will involve investigating your own requirements, the job market and the situations you are applying for.

The employer needs to be sure of her requirements; to identify where candidates with the right qualities can be found; and to assess their claims to have what is required. Perhaps less obvious is the need to investigate what might attract and retain them – that is, to investigate the candidate's needs. In a seller's market, this should not be overlooked.

If you are familiar with the notion of clinical investigation, you will realise that a systematic, thorough and critical approach is needed. This book will provide you with plenty of guidance to the right diagnosis.

Marketing

You will need to market yourself as a candidate, on paper and in person. The employer will need to market the organisation and the post on offer, and also herself as a colleague or boss.

Both employer and candidate need to consider their presentation to each other, to ensure that their meeting will be worthwhile. If you work as a nurse, you will have had to develop presentation skills in your work – for example, in presenting facts and ideas to colleagues. You may not have seen this as the basis for developing your interview style – but it could well be.

Matching

Although the interview itself is always seen as a process of selection for the employer, who has set it up to assess candidates, the candidate does also of course make an assessment of employers. This choice is going to be of increasing importance from now on. The matching process may also involve negotiation, to ensure that each party's needs are going to be met.

Matching implies that criteria have been set, against which a person or a job can be matched. Again, this should not be unfamiliar territory for people in clinical practice involved in assessment.

Evaluation

Evaluation is the outcome of a systematic matching process, based on objective criteria. It should be basically a rational decision, although most would allow some scope for intuition at times. Instead of evaluating a person's suitability for discharge or rehabilitation, for example, you will be evaluating whether your needs will be met by the job.

Evaluation is a two-way process, in that both parties will make judgements about whether the other party is offering what they want. If the quest is unsuccessful, then either side may want to ask why, in order to do better next time.

This book is about doing all of these things better, whether as a candidate or an interviewer. For the next 12 chapters, however, we shall be taking the candidate's part.

REFERENCE

Conroy, Margaret and Stidston, Mary, *2001 – The Black Hole – An Examination of Labour Market Trends in Relation to the NHS* (NHS Regional Manpower Planners' Group, 1988).

FURTHER READING

Herriott, P, *Recruitment in the 90s* (IPM, 1989).
Roberts, Celia, *The Interview Game and How It's Played* (BBC, 1985).

Chapter 2

MAKING A JOB CHANGE

To pursue the unattainable is insanity, yet the thoughtless can never refrain from doing so.   Marcus Aurelius, *Meditations*

A moment's insight is sometimes worth a life's experience.
    Oliver Wendell Holmes

WHY THINGS CANNOT BE THE SAME AFTERWARDS

In 'The day of judgement – the initiation', Sally had a choice. She decided that she wanted a new job. In her mind, she saw herself working in a new situation. In some way or other, in her mind at least, she left behind her current work situation, and got used to the idea of making a break with the here and now.

If she is offered the job, and accepts it, she will have to change, to adapt to a new situation. If she has not anticipated what she will be coming into, she is likely to be unhappy, and may regret the change. If she were to decide not to accept the offer, then she has to readjust to her current situation; if she had written it off for 'better things', there will be some disappointment. She will probably see herself as having outgrown her current job.

If she was seeking to escape from the frustrations of her current job, she will face the pain of having to get used to them again, possibly with a little humiliation at her failure. She will probably be going 'back to the drawing board' in terms of her escape strategy, to be sure of success next time.

It is important to realise this before you start the process of application. Even if you have no choice but to apply for a new job, because you are out of work or face redundancy, your feelings and self-image are put on the line. You may learn a lot, but equally, you may get hurt. In a thorough and demanding selection process, your failure is likely to come home to you heavily.

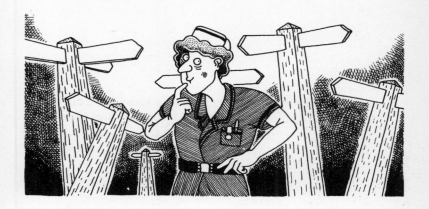

If the process you are subjected to seems weak and arbitrary, you may end up feeling angry with the interviewers, for not picking up what you had to offer. So often, though, failure leaves people with an empty feeling – not knowing what to think, because they did not know why they did not succeed. In Chapter 13, we will consider how you can obtain helpful feed-back. Sometimes the feedback is that the candidate 'failed to convince us' that she was the right person for the job. This is often seen by candidates as a failure of their presentation – to which the interviewee actor's response is often to work out a better interview script and delivery. In many cases, though, it is perhaps a perceptive panel telling the candidate that she has not really thought things through properly; that the application has been impulsive; or that there are likely to be problems that the candidate does not seem to have addressed.

Many organisations are not very good at selection, yet they are hungry to find talent. They will not have your interests at heart when they appoint you to a job that you went for on im-pulse. You may feel frustrated where you are, and be flattered at being given a new opportunity. However, it will not take you long to find out that it is not what you want.

So, the first lesson seems to be to know what you want.

KNOW WHAT YOU WANT

You are bound to want some security in your life; probably you will want some rewarding social networks, and to be able to pursue the things that give you satisfaction and fulfilment. People's ideas of security will differ. One person might put more importance on being a valued member of a working team, even if she could earn more elsewhere. Another person may see work as simply a means of making as much money as she can in order to leave and raise a family – or raise horses. In other words, some work to live and others live to work.

The job a person does is important, but may not be the most important thing in her life, or the most important way of meeting important needs. We need to be aware of our own needs very clearly, and they are changing all the time:

I thought I wanted more responsibility at one time – now I'm not so sure.

My children take up so much of my time, I really just want a job that means I can be with them as much as possible.

Now the children are off my hands, I would like to pursue my career again.

Professional needs

As a qualified nurse, you will have certain expectations about working as a professional. These will change over time. You may feel that things are going well, and that you simply want to develop the confidence and find the opportunity to fulfil your vocation fully:

I like nursing – it is the right career for me, but I just need to know how to develop my talents.

This might of course involve a change of job, as well as promotion:

I am not getting the satisfaction that I used to from nursing. Do I need to change direction?

Getting in touch with your expectations

You may want to reflect on what your expectations are, and

16

whether they are changing, or whether it is the job that has changed. Have you outgrown your current environment? Do you need some fresh challenges? Or merely a change of surroundings to reactivate your interest? You need to be clear whether the problem is with the setting you are working in; with the kind of nursing you are doing; with the level of responsibility you have; or with your feelings about clinical work, which may have changed. You may want to consider moving into management, or out of the NHS, or into a different clinical specialty, back into education, or out of nursing altogether.

THE DIAGNOSIS

Ask yourself the questions:

- What have been the high spots in my career so far?
- Where do I get my kicks?

Concentrate on what you've enjoyed most and where you've achieved most. What does your response tell you about:

- your capabilities?
- your ambitions?
- your values?
- factors affecting your self-confidence?
- the conditions where you will do best?

Think about all of your experiences so far, including those during your training. Think about the work itself, and also about the conditions you had to work in and the contact you had with others. Would you still find those experiences as rewarding, or have you moved on in some way?

Once you have a list of the things that motivate you positively, you might like to reflect on situations that were not so good, where you failed or were rather bored.

Should you re-evaluate some of your past experiences?

Would you cope with the down side any better now? Do you have some mental blocks about certain kinds of work because you handled it badly, through inexperience, or because you yourself were handled badly? Or has your past impression confirmed that certain things are not for you? Here is a checklist of the areas you should be considering.

Checklist 2.1

1 What you are good at.	What you are not good at.
2 What you enjoy.	What you don't enjoy.
3 Strengths.	Weaknesses/development
4 What you might need to	needs.
reconsider.	
5 How you are changing your	
interests and ideas.	

The following example shows what the checklist might look like when completed.

Example

1 What I'm good at:
- *Counselling*
- *Clinically demanding cases*
- *Teaching learners*

2 What I enjoy:
- *High-dependency patients*
- *Clinically demanding cases*
- *Teaching*

3 Strengths:
- *Clinical skills*
- *Counselling skills*
- *Teaching*

4 What I might need to reconsider:
- *A need to come to terms with administration*
- *Working with people I don't get on with*

What I'm not good at:
- *Routine administration*
- *Dealing with difficult people*
- *Working with people I don't get on with*

What I don't enjoy:
- *Administration*
- *Ward reports*
- *Drug administration*

Weaknesses/development needs:
- *Getting bored if not using skills*
- *Paperwork*
- *Oncology experience*

When you have your list, you might like to apply the following questions to it:

● Is there more on the 'plus' side than on the 'minus' side?
● Is there a pattern in your pluses? Or in your minuses?
● Does the pattern suggest that you have got some strong clinical interests? Or does it suggest that you are getting more from social contacts or the non-clinical side of the work?

Jane Schober has provided a checklist that you might find useful to focus your likes and dislikes.

Checklist 2.2

1 Which clinical specialty do you enjoy working in?
2 What type of work do you find most rewarding? For instance, do you prefer acute care, rehabilitation, involvement with patients and relatives, or teaching patients?
3 Do you prefer working in a unit, in a ward or in the community?
4 Do you enjoy being busy at work?
5 Do you thrive on responsibility? For example, do you like being in charge or being a team leader?
6 Do you prefer to work as a member of a team, or independently, as health visitors and district nurses do?

Taking stock of the skills you have

Which of the skills given in the following checklist have you demonstrated in your work, or in your life generally? You may think of others.

Checklist 2.3

1 Clinical skills (in which areas?):
   - practice
   - setting policy
   - assessment/evaluation.
2 Skills with people:
   - counselling
   - teaching
   - conducting interviews
   - negotiating
   - relaxing people
   - giving support
   - relating to children.
3 Organising skills:
   - analysing and solving problems
   - setting up systems
   - maintaining records
   - financial management
   - planning projects
   - getting things sorted out
   - household management.
4 Leadership skills:
   - taking initiatives
   - team building
   - taking-charge skills
   - persuading and encouraging others
   - directing others
   - running meetings
   - providing inspiration.
5 Technical skills:
   - handling equipment
   - repairing things
   - design and construction
   - mathematical calculations
   - research
   - clinical or other teaching
   - designing learning
   - assessment
   - computing
   - cooking
   - childrearing skills
   - other practical skills like sewing, typing or gardening.
6 Communication skills:
   - speaking
   - writing.

Note those that are definitely a strong point, or those that you would like to develop, as well as those that are of little interest to you or have little potential for you.

As a nurse, you will have had to use very many of these skills in one way or another. If there are particular skills that you enjoy using, you may want to seek the opportunity to develop them further. In some cases, a job that offers you no scope for developing them might be frustrating.

Once you have taken stock of the skills you have, you might also reveal some skills that you could use outside of nursing, if you wanted to. Consequently, in a nursing interview, you will be confident that you can sell yourself as having these skills, in addition to the clinical ones.

Places you might like to have been to

Are you conscious that you have *not* had certain experiences, which might have been rewarding for you? Perhaps you have stayed within a particular specialty, or within the ward or theatres, or in one hospital, or in hospital as opposed to the community? Is there a 'somewhere else' that attracts you? If so, how much do you know about it? Are you likely to be able to put your talents to good use? What motivations are required? Are they your motivations?

You may have seen a job advertisement that looks interesting. Try to imagine what it would be like to do that job – and imagine the possible drawbacks. Do not just think about the work. Think about having further to travel, having to make new friends, or possibly moving house.

Here is another checklist – this time of reasons for wanting to change your job. I have added some cautionary notes – forgive me for playing the concerned parent.

Checklist 2.4

1 Are you interested in developing your career at present?
... even if it may not be your most pressing concern, identify whether you might change your mind later. Not everyone has to be a careerist.

2 Do you think you are ready for promotion?
... this supposes a 'yes' to question 1, and your diagnosis should reveal this – but do your bosses and advisers agree? Are you mistaking frustration for ambition?

3 Are you stressed at work?
... if so, do you know why? Have you given the job a fair trial, or discussed the stresses with anyone at work? By acting impetuously, you might be jumping from the frying pan into the fire.

4 Have you lost interest in your current job?
... try to establish the reasons for this. It may be that your efforts are not being properly rewarded, or that you have developed new interests. Discussion with colleagues might help change things or open new doors for you.

5 Do you need to do a course of study?
... have you considered which course and your reasons for this choice? If it is simply escapism or the desire for a new stimulus, be sure that you are jumping in the right direction.

6 Do you want to leave the health authority for personal or social reasons – such as family reasons – or because the cost of living is too high where you are?
... are there other, less drastic solutions to your problems? Think what you might lose if you got out.

7 Have you developed an interest in another area of nursing?
... do you know enough about it, or are you simply copying other people or doing what seems fashionable?

8 Are you facing a ward or unit closure?
... are you aware of your rights and of the help your employer must give you? It might be an opportunity in disguise.

9 Are all of your friends and contemporaries getting out? Is sister getting on your nerves?
... not good enough I am afraid!

10 Do you want to get away from household chores and childminding but are anxious about being out of date?
... do you know about preparatory courses being run by many colleges these days, including clinical updating and study skills?

The lessons here are:

1 Be clear about why you need to move.
2 Have a plan. Do not act on impulse or you may genuinely regret it.
3 It helps to have someone with whom you can discuss your career.

Can you now put down an answer to the question 'Where are you going?'. How about the 'How will you get there?' question? There may be several routes to be considered, as illustrated in the following case studies.

Case study 1

Julie Brandt has been a ward sister for two years in the London teaching hospital in which she trained. She staffed for two years before her promotion. She is happy in her job, but wants to teach eventually and is not sure whether she ought to seek experience elsewhere first, and, if so, where and in what field. Her current post is in a gynaecology ward. Julie needs to consider several options. If she wants to qualify as a nurse tutor, she will need to fulfil the UKCC criteria relating to her statutory qualification, professional experience and evidence of professional knowledge.

Her experience as a ward sister is valuable; there does not appear to be a need to change post unless she feels that she would benefit from further clinical or managerial experience.

Prospective nurse teachers must have completed a course of study beyond statutory qualification, which should normally not be less than six months full-time. Such courses include the diploma in nursing and nursing degree courses. Julie would be advised to seek advice from the director of nurse education at her hospital, who would be able to advise her of possible opportunities and explain the UKCC criteria.

In the meantime, Julie might consider undertaking a short teaching course such as the English National Board (ENB) course 998 'Teaching and assessing in clinical practice', which is run in many schools of nursing as a way of developing teaching skills relevant to her clinical area. The course also offers theoretical input, which would give her the opportunity to judge her reasons for wishing to enter teaching.

Case study 2

After qualifying, Angela Smythe staffed for six months at her training hospital – a district general hospital – then took a staff nurse's post in another hospital.

Three years later she was promoted to sister in a men's medical ward. She has been in the post for two and a half years. Angela feels on top of her job now and is ready for a move. She has no family ties and no special career aspirations.

Angela has several options. She can stay where she is and develop her post under the direction and guidance of her nurse manager. This might include developing patient allocation systems, for example, or primary nursing, teaching in the ward or undertaking a research project.

If Angela is ready for a move, she would need to assess her reasons for this, her areas of interest and the potential benefits of such a move. This may take the form of a course of study. Possibly she would be able to combine a part-time course with a full-time job. A course relevant to nursing, such as an ENB clinical course or a course in research (ENB 995), would be useful if she wants to remain in clinical nursing. A course at certificate, diploma or degree level, relevant to nursing, would facilitate entry into teaching.

Case study 3

Denise Ryan is a staff nurse with seven years' experience in medical wards. When her hospital closed, she explored all of the options open to her in other local hospitals, and finally decided that she would like to train for the community as a district nurse. This was an option she had been considering for some time but had not actively pursued. The conditions of the authority's re-deployment agreement meant that she could be sponsored for this, if accepted for training.

Figure 2.1 summarises the steps involved in making a job change.

FURTHER READING

Details of ENB courses, certificate, diploma and degree courses for clinical nurses and prospective nurse teachers may be obtained from the ENB careers office. If you are considering a post abroad, it is advisable to contact the RCN International Department and the UKCC. Some useful addresses are given in Appendix 3.

Baker, Jill, *What Next?* (Macmillan, 1988).

Bolles, Richard N, *What Color is Your Parachute?* (Ten Speed Press, USA, 1987).

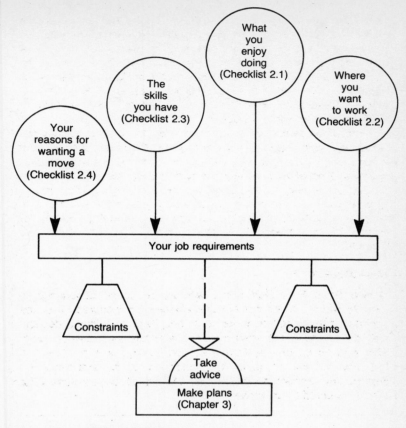

Figure 2.1 *Job change summary chart*

DH Nursing Division Career Development Project Group, *The Way Ahead: Career Pathways for Nurses, Midwives and Health Visitors* (Department of Health, 1988).

Golzen, G and Plumbley, P, *Changing Your Job after 35*, 6th Edn (Kogan Page, 1985).

Lancashire, Ruth and Holdsworth, Roger, *Career Change* (Hobson's Press, 1976).

Truman, Carole, *Overcoming the Career Break: A Positive Approach* (Manpower Services Commission, 1986).

Tschudin, Verena, *Managing Yourself*, Essentials of Nursing Management series (Macmillan, 1990).

Willis, Margaret, *Job Hunting for Women* (Kogan Page, 1987).

Chapter 3

TARGETING THE OPPORTUNITY

A wise man will make more opportunities than he finds.

Francis Bacon

FINDING JOBS

Checking out the advertisements

Let us suppose that you have done your preliminary work and considered the net benefits to you of making a change, taking account of personal, professional and social factors. You are now looking through the appointments columns.

Most professional workers do not need to be told where to look for job advertisements. You know what you want and there will be dozens of employers keen to tell you that they have it.

Is it a fashionable specialty, or a famous hospital? Make sure that you are not blinded by the glamorous image. You may know people who work in the place, who can give you a balanced picture. If not, you will have to find out for yourself.

Employers like to give you the impression that they are offering the most up-to-date facilities, conditions and care policies in their advertising. But do not be misled by attractive packaging. In the light of fierce competition, personnel and nurse managers pay a lot more attention now to promoting their image, and writing copy for job ads that is sometimes misleading. The worst thing that can happen is that both employer and employee oversell themselves to each other, resulting in a dreadful mismatch and disillusionment.

Getting information from contacts

You may need to update yourself, or talk to an expert, about the latest practice in a particular specialty. You need to be able to identify the signs of high standards and a progressive approach to care, both from what is said on paper and from your visit.

You will probably find it quite easy to get in touch with a 'friend of a friend' who knows the specialty or place you are interested in. One of the benefits of working in nursing is the access you have to a wide range of helpful contacts. If friends cannot help, ask tutors, or your union steward. Be persistent. The employer may not tell you, in the glossy package that you are sent, that accommodation is unavailable, awful or too expensive; that the shops are five miles away and public transport is poor; that the staff crèche facilities are not quite what they might seem; that the health and safety standards are inadequate; or that there is risk of violence on the A & E department at night.

Most NHS health districts issue a regular internal vacancy bulletin. These sometimes cover vacancies in neighbouring health districts.

You may hear of jobs through your network of friends and contacts. You may know where there are developments taking place, and it is well worth making enquiries. Ring up the unit personnel office or unit nursing office. Of course, if the place where you are interested in working is still being built, it will not be obvious where to ring for information. In such cases, check which health district (or private health organisation) is involved and ask their headquarters personnel office for the number and address of the recruitment office. Most recruiters will be happy to take your details and send you full information when it becomes available. However, there is no point in applying more than six months before a place opens.

Occasionally, jobs will be advertised in local papers. This is much cheaper than in the professional journals, and will some-times attract one or two staff nurses living locally for jobs in medical or surgical areas.

Speculative calls

You may like to make a few speculative telephone calls to places you like the look of. Hospitals and health centres rarely have no vacancies these days, so this may be worthwhile. The addresses and telephone numbers given in the *Nursing Times* job advertisements will be the ones to ring for information about vacancies. Do not ring the nurse manager quoted unless you are prepared to be quizzed about your reasons for leaving your current job and your experience to date. This kind of enquiry will be discussed later in the chapter. If anyone asks you why you are enquiring, say you are interested in seeking work in the area and thought that the place in question might be one where you might like to work. If you prefer to write a letter on these lines, enclose a stamped addressed envelope. The letter may well be placed on a file; the telephone enquiry may get lost.

Before you start job hunting in earnest, if may be useful to identify clearly what you want. The following checklist is designed for this purpose.

Checklist 3.1

1 The post:
   Note down the kinds of post you are interested in: grade, specialty, kind of job; salary, hours, shift arrangements, including weekend working. Note also the particular requirements you need from a job.

2 The geography:
   Note where you might want to work (and perhaps where not), in terms of geographical area, access to transport, pleasant countryside, housing, etc.

3 The work location:
   Do the same in terms of hospital or centre, work setting, size of clinical unit, facilities available, learning and development opportunities, etc. Note any possible security or access problems.

4 The employer:
   What extras are important to you? Opportunities for further training and promotion is an obvious one, and so is staff accommodation. What about recreational facilities on site? The chance of a lease car being offered, if you have to travel? You can change your mind later if necessary, but focusing on what is important *before* you start looking will help you to assess what is being offered more clearly in relation to your own wants.

5 Your networks:
   Think of people you know who might be useful contacts in

---

your job search: people in those parts of the country, or specialties, where you might like to work; people, for example tutors, who are likely to be in the know about a lot of things, or to know other people whom you can get in touch with; someone who has worked in a particular place, or even one who has been for an interview there once, or who has worked in that specialty.

The following example identifies the requirements of three nurses and shows what the checklist might look like when completed.

Example

Requirement	Nurse 1	Nurse 2	Nurse 3
The post	D grade Preferably medical Nights or 3 days/week	E grade Normal hours Preferably alternate weekends	H grade Community
The geography	Near home	South of England	Within 10 miles of current home
The work location	1 of 3 local hospitals	Prefer teaching hospital Good social life Cheap accommodation	Rural preferred
The employer	Must give some flexibility during holidays	Opportunities for study required	Further training for management

WHAT YOU CAN TELL FROM ADVERTISEMENTS

NHS advertisements in the professional press usually conform to rigid guidelines on their layout. Occasionally, they can have a more personalised style.

The design can tell you how important the post might be to the employer. If the advertisement takes up half or a full page, the employer is very keen to attract your attention, possibly because she is chronically short of staff in a particular service.

Advertisements give employers the chance to tell you something about themselves. If they are taking recruitment seriously, the text should be of high quality. A good advertisement will tell you exactly where posts are based, a little about the service, and something of the social and living environment. It should also tell you who to contact for further details. A general advertisement for staff nurses, which gives scant details of the areas on offer, needs careful scrutiny.

Take care to read how the employer has presented the contact point. An advertiser who tells you to phone Miss C Littlechurch is not exactly attempting to be friendly. A more informal approach would advise you to contact Carol Littlechurch and tell you what her job is. Some may be very informal and invite you to contact Carol, personnel officer, for a chat. Simple signals can be picked up by reading with care.

Outside the NHS, the range and style of advertisements vary enormously.

Job titles can also be important in an advertisement. Mary Jones had applied for a job described as 'matron on a university campus'. The job involved running a mini-centre for first aid and a sick bay for staff and students in the halls of residence. The advertisement had not referred to a salary. One nurse, presuming that the salary would be based on NHS nursing scales, was slack in checking details. After she had held the job for some months, she discovered that she was not on any NHS nursing scale, but on ancillary scales, which applied in the education field, and thus national NHS pay rises did not apply to her.

The advertisement can only provide a brief picture of the post and employer. You may well be invited to apply for an application form and information pack so that you can find out more. If an employer is not prepared to provide an information pack, it may reveal a complacent attitude to recruitment.

The quality of the information pack can also tell you a lot about the employer. A well-designed, well-written and well-presented pack shows that some thought has been given to what is likely to attract staff. For instance, a good employer will provide detailed information about the cost and quality of local accommodation and leisure and social amenities.

A good information pack should be factual about all aspects of the job and employment. A good employer will not let potential applicants base important decisions on erroneous information. The following checklist shows what to look for.

Checklist 3.2

1 The advertisement:
   Is it lively and engaging? Does it give a clear picture of the job, including:
   - What the job entails?
   - Whether the salary scale matches the job title?
   - What leisure and social amenities are available in the local area?
   - Whether accommodation is available?
   - Who to contact and what the person's name and job title is?

2 The information pack:
   An interested employer should provide one. Think twice about the job if it doesn't. Does it say something about the employer? Is the impression a smooth image with too much 'hype'? Or is it a shabby presentation? Does it indicate a concern for individuals?
   The pack should contain detailed information on:
   - The job (including grade, salary, hours and shifts).
   - The place of work.
   - The location, including leisure and social amenities.
   - Accommodation – the standard, cost and its proximity to the job.
   - Further training opportunities.
   - The requirements of people needed.
   - Details of the selection process.

MAKING DIRECT CONTACT

Perhaps you have found out all you can from what has been sent to you and from your contacts. You may have rejected those posts that seem to have critical limitations as far as you are concerned. You may have rejected others because they did not ring true, and you suspected they were being oversold.

The prowl visit

You may decide that you need more information about some posts. What can you do? You can use your contacts, if you have any. If you need to see the place, and you live or work nearby, you might at this stage like to make a 'prowl visit'. The idea is to take advantage of the fact that many hospitals and centres are open to the public and that they will not know who you are at this stage. If it is appropriate to visit the place – and sometimes it is not – go during visiting hours.

On a prowl visit, you can tell a lot just from superficial impressions:

- The general appearance and state of decorations. Is it neglected and impoverished, or well cared for and well endowed?
- Is it congested or spacious?
- Is it well equipped or is equipment rather sparse and outmoded?
- Is it busy? Do there seem to be enough staff?
- Is there a friendly atmosphere?
- Is it isolated or right in the hub of things?
- Do you feel secure there?
- Is it too hot or too cold?

Contact by telephone

You may need to make direct contact with the person named in the advertisement to check on one or two things, and possibly arrange an informal visit. Since this is the first direct contact you will make, our second consideration, that of (self) *presentation*, is relevant here. You should know what you are going to ask before you pick up the telephone. Note it down.

You may have to give your name, and therefore any impression you give may be remembered. They may want to ask you about yourself, if you say you are interested in applying.

The first impression you give must be a favourable one. You are not yet ready to present yourself to them. Here are some examples of what you don't want to happen:

- You ring up and say that you have the details of the job but that there is nothing about secondment for ENB courses, and that is your main reason for applying. If you do not show interest in the job itself, they will not be impressed.
- You ring up and say you are interested in applying. You ask what sort of experience they are looking for. Rather than get the answers you want, an insistent nurse manager asks you all sorts of questions and the conversation begins to feel like a telephone interview that you have not prepared for. You must avoid getting drawn in at this early stage.
- When you try to ask about the quality of clinical care, they

say 'Why do you want to know?' in a rather suspicious tone. You have to get information without putting them on the defensive.

Here then is some general guidance:

1   Find out about them and also about what they want.
    You will probably want to find out more about them and their job, as well as what they are seeking in applicants. The latter is more difficult.
2   Express interest in the job.
    Always start off by saying that you've seen the advertisement and it looks like a very interesting job. Mention some clinical aspect that seems particularly good. Let the person talk about it. Then ask if they have a minute or so to answer one or two of your questions before you decide to make an application.
3   Be prepared to say a little about yourself.
    Although you would do well to avoid it at this stage, you may need to be prepared to say a little about your interests and background – but do not get dragged into a telephone interview.
4   Do not let yourself be interviewed.
    If there is a danger of this, say 'Well, naturally, I will be sending you full details of my background if and when I apply, so I'd rather not go into detail now.' If you want to know what they are looking for, it is better to ask direct questions, like 'How many months' experience are you seeking as a minimum?' or 'Will you accept a recently qualified nurse for this post?' rather than 'I don't think I have much experience. Do you think I would have any chance of being shortlisted?' If you do that, they are bound to start asking you how much experience you have, and start to interview you.
5   Do not expect the whole truth about everything.
    It is unlikely that some questions will be answered truthfully, like 'Do you have high standards?', 'Why did the last person leave?', 'Are you finding it difficult to get staff?', 'Will I get good training in your department?' or even 'What exactly are you looking for?'.
6   Be subtle in your questions.
    You may get some idea of the answers you want by being a little bit more oblique: 'Are you planning to introduce such

33

and such a technique?' (which you know is the most recent work in the field); 'I expect it's difficult to keep staff, as once they have some experience they are in demand elsewhere' (do they encourage development and internal promotion?); 'I have noticed a lot of advertisements for these posts in the past two months. Are you expanding the service?'; 'I expect you get a lot of applicants with such and such experience.'

7 Be polite and show enthusiasm.

If you want to probe, you must do it politely; and if your questions are in fact somewhat mercenary, you will need to convey some enthusiasm for the work at the same time. Thank the person for taking the trouble to answer your questions. You may want to indicate whether you are likely to apply, or whether 'It is not really what I want'. Make sure you are clear about how the selection is to be carried out.

If you are able to make a positive contact, you may well agree on the telephone to make an informal visit. Make sure you get the name of the person you are speaking to on the telephone. She may turn out to be a 'friend' later on. Give yourself a day or two to prepare for this visit. You will be able to make further investigations at that stage, but you will also need to consider your presentation. Before you think about whether you need a new outfit for this, you need to know more about what they are looking for. We will go into this in the next chapter.

Figure 3.1 summarises the steps involved in finding a job.

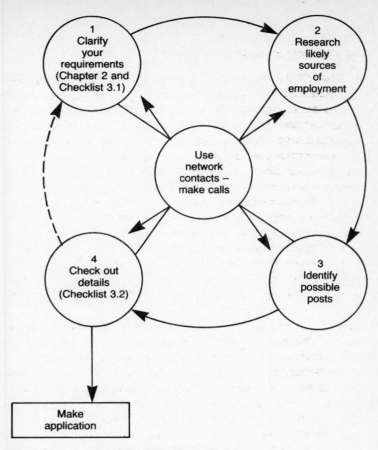

Figure 3.1 *Job finding summary chart*

Chapter 4

THE INFORMAL VISIT

WHY AN INFORMAL VISIT?

It is generally wise to take up the offer of an informal visit if you are seriously considering the job. If you cannot visit because of the distance, explain in writing and ask for a visit to be arranged at the time of your interview.

Ask, if possible, if you can visit the actual place of work, and maybe talk to the staff as well as the manager. Any hesitation in allowing you to do this may tell you something about the place.

Some employers are concerned that informal visits will give candidates some opportunity to influence the outcomes of interviews, which will be unfair on those who cannot attend. To avoid this, a visit to the work setting may be offered as part of the interview arrangements.

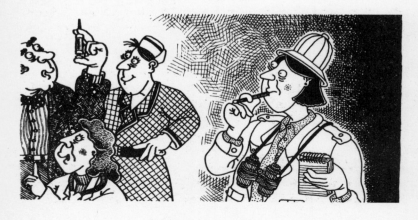

An informal visit is not an interview. Ideally, it should be conducted by someone who has nothing to do with the interview process. However, the person who will be most useful to you in explaining what happens will be the manager who is recruiting for the post, and you may well want to meet this person in an informal setting. It is also very probable that she will be taking part in the interview arrangements.

Unless advertised as such, your visit should not be allowed to become a situation where they interview you, but rather a chance for you to find out about them and what they are looking for.

PREPARATION

Study the information pack before you go. This will enable you to ask some relevant questions, giving the impression of someone who is well-informed, or who has done her homework. You should identify the information you still need from the checklists in Chapter 3.

You will probably want to find out what kind of person they are looking for, and as much as you can about local conditions and practices. There may be a chance to ask about the locality and accommodation, as well as training facilities.

HOW TO BEHAVE

Be prepared for some scrutiny by the staff and managers concerned. Hence, your appearance and demeanour do matter on a visit. If you are visiting a drop-in centre for drug abusers, it is reasonable to assume that dress will not be too formal. If, on the other hand, you are visiting an up-market private clinic or a hospital-based environment, you will probably need to dress more formally.

You will be concerned to put yourself across as friendly and polite, and interested in the job. Show yourself to be a good listener, and smile and ask questions. If you want time to talk, you should visit during the early evening, rather than at the busiest part of the day.

MEET THOSE WORKING THERE

You may want to meet staff working in the area you are considering, particularly those on a similar grade to the post for which you are applying. You can safely ask them to give you an honest picture of the work setting, mentioning some of the bad as well as good things. Ask them how long they have been working there.

Be suspicious if the person you have come to see is reluctant for you to talk to people, or wants to control what you see. Do not be afraid to ask to see things. Your interest and friendliness will be noted, and will not usually be seen as nosiness. However, do not outstay your welcome. It is inevitable that all of your reactions to things will be noted, and possibly reported to others, so do not get carried away. Be enthusiastic but restrained.

WHAT TO LOOK OUT FOR

Is there a good atmosphere in the place? Is it formal or informal? Is it friendly to visitors? Do people seem to know what they are doing? Are there enough staff? Do they get on with each other, have a sense of humour? Is it a pleasant physical environment? Do nursing standards seem high? Is the equipment up to date and plentiful, and in working order? You will often get better answers to these types of query by observing for yourself, rather than by asking questions.

Look at how people relate to each other on your visit. You may find the place is like a palace, but, if nobody smiles or relationships seem totally formal and rigid, would you be happy working there?

They may be wary of giving you too many clues that you can use later in your self-presentation at the formal interview. You will almost certainly get some idea of their enthusiasm for your application, and they will be assessing whether or not you might 'fit in' socially. If you are too outspoken or critical, obviously they will feel defensive and may jump to the conclusion that you are likely to cause problems for them. On the other hand, do not be mouselike either. Do not be afraid to ask questions. Besides the useful information you will obtain, you will get an idea of the receptiveness of the managers to your queries, and may give the impression of someone with clear ideas and confidence.

If you are really put off, you may want to tell them that it is not really what you are looking for, there and then. If, on the other hand, you feel some enthusiasm for working there, you will be motivated to prepare thoroughly for the interview itself.

AVOIDING BEING GRILLED

Remember that the visit is provided simply to give you an insight into the post you are applying for; you should not be grilled about your knowledge at this time. Such areas should be discussed only at interview, and the informal visit should not be abused.

If people are showing signs of asking too much about your own background, you might indicate that you are anxious to be somewhere else. Make your apologies and assure them that you will be sure to give them full details if you decide to apply. If you feel that they have abused the situation, you may not want to anyway. It is as well to be aware of the fact that some employers see nothing wrong in using the informal visit as an opportunity to do some informal screening of candidates. If you are taken by surprise, say 'I'm sorry, but I am afraid I am not ready to take part in an interview right now.'

Some employers will use the pretext of giving you advice to assess whether you seem to be the right person for the job, often subtly prefaced by 'Do you think this is what you are looking for?'. It is best to say 'possibly', and not to get drawn into a discussion, unless that is what you want.

What you say about yourself, and the impression you give, must match what you say in the application form or CV (curriculum vitae). You must remember what you have said about yourself and reinforce this when you apply.

The following checklist will help you to prepare for an informal visit.

Checklist 4.1

1   Preparation:
    - Study the information pack.
    - Identify what you need to know.
    - Prepare questions you want to ask.
    - Visit outside of busy periods.
2   How to behave:
    - Be prepared to be scrutinised.
    - Be friendly and polite.
    - Be a good listener.
    - React positively.
    - Do not be critical.
    - Do not outstay your welcome.

---

3   Meet the workers:
    - Find out how they feel.
4   What to look out for:
    - The atmosphere.
    - The staffing.
    - The relationships.
    - The equipment.
    - The conditions.
    - The receptions to you.
    - Note what you are not shown.

Chapter 5

PRESENTING YOURSELF ON PAPER

What is written without effort is in general read without pleasure.
Dr Samuel Johnson

SETTING OUT YOUR STALL – AN ANALOGY

You have seen the advertisement for the job you want, you have 'done a prowl' and obtained further information, now you want to apply for it.

Your application is the first formal step towards obtaining your new job and – unlike preliminary forays – is a permanent record, which is likely not only to be seen but judged.

You are now entering the job market and setting out your stall. How you do it will either attract people towards buying what you have to offer – your talents or skills – or put them off. So, it is only common sense to arrange your wares so that they catch the eye and draw in customers. This is an inappropriate time to indulge in the nursing habit of self-depreciation.

We all know how magnetic a well-arranged stall can be. To carry the analogy a little further, it is often the display of just one special attraction that excites the customer. A little later in this chapter, we discuss how to highlight aspects of your career to attract the prospective employer. First, we concentrate on setting up the stall itself.

PREPARATION

Applying for the job you want is not something to be done in the odd five-minute tea-break. If you are to do yourself justice, you will need to take time and make an effort to present yourself well.

The personal dossier

At the beginning of your career, you are not likely to be asked to produce a CV, but rather to complete an application form. Nevertheless, it is a good idea to prepare a personal record for yourself. Not only is it an excellent opportunity to really think about what you have done up to now, it also provides you with a permanent record of your achievements.

As time goes by, you will have done more, learned more, taken responsibility for different areas, attended courses, and so on. Remembering all of these things is difficult. It will be extremely frustrating for you if, like some people, you have to rummage through the accumulated papers of a lifetime to find the attendance record for a professional development course that you completed two (or maybe three?) years ago.

Start now, if you haven't already, to keep a personal dossier of events in your working life. Put down dates, including short notes on what you have done, and attach relevant papers to it.

You can add to your dossier the skills and competencies referred to in Chapter 2. Do not forget the skills you have acquired that are not directly related to nursing. Women and men who run a household while bringing up a family have, of necessity, to become good at budgeting, negotiation and compromise (toddlers can give politicians lessons in intransigence), not to mention teaching and time management.

Added to these skills may be interpersonal skills you have acquired in committee work or group activities outside work, for clubs and voluntary organisations, for schools and pressure groups. These skills are of no less importance than those used in the workplace. Do not underestimate yourself – but do not overestimate either.

Be honest. If you have faults, gaps in your knowledge or skeletons in your cupboard, you should be aware of them. Chapter 8 deals with such problems in greater detail.

Your personal dossier will help you with applications for jobs, and will act as a useful *aide-mémoire* when you are preparing for an interview. It will also help you to anticipate the interviewer's questions and formulate intelligent questions yourself. What did you learn on that professional development course? Will you have opportunities to use your knowledge in this or that job?

Once you have started your dossier, you will need to update it as new experiences occur.

Getting down to it

Once you have gathered all the necessary information, you should set aside a quiet time to complete your application. You have three goals to achieve in preparing your written application which will secure you the interview for the job you want:

1 appearance
2 completeness and relevance
3 the 'special offer'.

The first two goals will be discussed here, but a discussion of the 'special offer' will be left to later in the chapter.

Appearance

It should go without saying that your application should be neatly and legibly written in blue or black ink, or typed, and accompanied by a short letter.

Employers judge on appearances. We may deplore the typical snap judgements made – for example, you do not need to be able to spell in order to be a good nurse – nonetheless there is a grain of truth in the assumption that a person who sends in a scruffy application form may also make a mess of the patients' notes.

It would be a pity to lose the chance of an interview through carelessness.

Completeness and relevance

Although you will want to highlight some aspects of your experience (we discuss this later), you should not miss out long periods of your life, or put down false information. People experienced in reading application forms and CVs will have their suspicions aroused if you do.

If you have skipped from job to job, or have other skeletons to conceal, you may indeed have problems. (Chapter 8 gives further advice.) Leaving blanks on the application form invites questions: it could be seen as carelessness, something you want to hide, or it may even be read as an unwelcome indication of your openness or attitude to enquiries.

Standard application forms will ask you to list your previous posts. Make sure you do it in the required order. CVs should also include details of all previous posts.

The employer will note that you have acquired some skills in all of these jobs, and she will be seeking evidence of progression, particularly if it is a career post for which you are applying. Assisting with a playgroup, for example, would be worth mentioning, as it shows that you are keen on organising or relating to others.

THE APPLICATION FORM

Most health service jobs up to middle management level will require you to complete a standard application form. Although the style differs from authority to authority, each contains a comon core of questions, which you can answer easily enough using your own personal dossier. Chapter 6 gives hints on choosing referees.

What makes you special?

You can fairly assume that most other candidates applying for the job will have the basic qualifications required. How do you make your application stand out from the crowd? The key element here is the little space left for 'additional information that you may think relevant'. This comes towards the end of the form, together perhaps with 'brief outline of current responsibilities'. On some forms, these may be combined. Here, you are being given the opportunity to sell your abilities in a few sentences. You must seize it! You can find out how to do so in a later section, headed 'the special offer'.

THE CV

For more senior jobs, and for those outside the health service, you may be asked to provide a CV, rather than to complete an application form.

The conventional CV is very simply a list of your personal

details and achievements, compiled by you, but providing much the same information as an application form.

Your CV should list your name, home address, telephone number, date of birth, sex and marital status. Next, you should list your qualifications, starting with basic nursing qualification, the date you received it and your UKCC registration number. This should be followed by the details of other post-basic nursing, health visiting or midwifery qualifications, if any. Include here any short certificated course you may have attended, or open-learning modules you may have completed.

Add any non-nursing qualifications that may be relevant. You will have to use your common sense here. A university degree is worth mentioning; fluency in Urdu would be of immense benefit in an inner city post but of little practical use in a rural area; a driving licence is a necessity for a community post; a hang-gliding instructor's certificate is of little relevance in nursing.

The CV should detail the posts you have held, starting with your current position. Give the month and year in which you started the job, and the month and year you left it. Set down the job title, followed by a short sentence describing the responsibilities you think worth mentioning. It must be short – do not be tempted into a lengthy explanation of every aspect of the job. The list should take you as far back as your student days. If you were awarded the gold medal, say so.

When you are compiling your employment record, do differentiate between jobs within the same hospital or health authority. If you have been promoted, or have moved into a different area for experience, then treat each as a separate job.

Next, list your publications, if any, and other relevant details, such as participation as a speaker at conferences, or attendance at local study days or uncertificated courses. If you are a member of your professional organisation, and any of its sub-groups, add these in here.

It is a matter of opinion whether to include outside interests within a CV. On one hand, your outside interests may be relevant to your career, in which case you should probably include them; or they may give a more rounded picture of you as a person, as well as offering a peg for conversation at the interview. On the other hand, some people find them an irrelevance in a professional CV. It is up to you to decide which way seems most relevant to the ambience of the organisation to which you are applying.

Finally, you should give the names of two people who are willing to act as referees (see Chapter 6 for further information).

Figure 5.1 shows a typical, conventional CV. Ideally, your CV should be typed. It is worth a box of chocolates to a competent typist to achieve this!

What makes you special?

Because you prepare it yourself, a CV provides an opportunity to depart from the conventional mode of presentation, if you feel it is appropriate to the job and the employer you are seeking. It is up to you to judge what is most suitable.

It is certainly the case that a new CV should be prepared for each job you apply for. Nothing is more likely to provide you with a curt rejection letter than to send a photocopy of a CV obviously prepared some time ago with additions in pen, or with a separate update sheet stapled on. Your CV should be newly prepared with one particular job in mind.

But it requires more than this to make your application stand out from the crowd. It is current practice, when you are asked to provide a CV, to preface it with a short (perhaps one side of paper) essay highlighting your particular relevant experience for the job. This has a number of advantages. It allows you to provide the conventional CV, while at the same time saying more about yourself. It shows prospective employers that you have taken the time and trouble to consider their requirements and how you match up to them. It gives them a reason for shortlisting you for interview, and offers a starting point for discussion at the interview, in which you can participate with some confidence.

You may be aware of gaps in your knowledge or defects in your CV. If you can accentuate the positive areas of your skill and experience, you may well, at the same time, diminish the effect of the negative ones. The next section examines how to do this.

The special offer

You have set up your stall in the market. Now comes the real sales ability – your first opportunity to sell yourself. You will need to consider carefully what you have learned about the job from the job specification provided by the employer, and if

Name: Claire Vickers
Address: 30 Old Lane, Bushwood, Sussex

Telephone No: 0127 82967, ext. 434 (daytime)
                       0217 46544 (after 7 p.m.)

Date of birth: September 24, 1961
Sex: Female
Marital status: Divorced, no children

Qualifications: RGN (1982) No: 22389757 Diploma in nursing
                         (1986)
                         ENB Intensive care course (1988)
                         Open university course in child health (1987)

Posts held:
March 1988—present: Staff nurse, ICU, Adams Hospital, Devon
                         Senior of eight staff nurses in 8-bed unit

May 1987—February 1988: Staff nurse (nights), orthopaedic
                         ward, Adams Hospital, Devon. In charge of
                         16-bed ward with teaching responsibilities

March 1985—March 1987: Staff nurse, orthopaedic ward,
                         Sheikh Al Kharam Hospital, Saudi Arabia

September 1982—March 1985: Staff nurse, general surgical
                         ward, St Lawrence's Hospital, Uttlesford

September 1979—September 1982: Nursing student,
                         St Lawrence's Hospital, Uttlesford

Publications: 'If you don't like the heat ...', *Nursing Times*,
                         June 1987

Professional organisation: RCN; member of the intensive
                         care nurse forum

Interests: Reading detective novels; show jumping

Referees: Miss P. Appleton   James D. Scrivenor
                   Sister   Director of Nursing Services
                   ICU   Adams Hospital
                   Adams Hospital   Plymouth, Devon.
                   Plymouth, Devon.
Please do not consult either referee unless I am shortlisted for
the post.

Figure 5.1   *The conventional CV*

you are lucky, from the person specification. If you have made an informal visit or a prowl, or simply spoken on the telephone, you will have more to add to your knowledge.

Next, try to take a broad view of yourself and what you have to offer, not only in terms of experience, but in terms of enthusiasm, personal qualities and ability to learn.

Now you must try to match up the two. You may find that the easiest way of doing this is to make a list of, say, six key elements of the job as described by the employer which you have spotted. Then, against each element, write down your own experience in that area (if none, write none).

Once you have completed the list, you should be in a position to judge which of all of your skills or experiences is likely to impress.

If you are completing an application form, it is perhaps best to choose just one or two items to mention in that 'further information' slot. For the preface sheet accompanying a CV, you may prefer to discuss briefly three or four elements that highlight your experience in different areas – clinical, management, teaching or interprofessional relationships, for example. If, on reflection, you seem to have just one particular relevant talent, then concentrate on that.

The following example shows how to set out these crucial sentences – and a few sentences are enough. You can expand on your experiences at the interview.

Example

In my current post, I enlisted the help of a visiting speech therapist in setting up a communications group for seven of our elderly psychiatric patients. This group now meets for half an hour daily with a nurse to act as co-ordinator and leader. While progress was initially slow, the patients are now showing real progress in their ability to communicate with each other, rather than through the nurses.

These few sentences will give an alert employer a number of clues as to your suitability for the job, as say, senior charge nurse, grade G in a psychiatric hospital.

Here is an analysis of what the employer sees in your sales pitch:

1 You are an innovator ('*I enlisted. . .*'). But if you have simply

been involved in someone else's innovation, then beware of claiming it for yourself. You may come unstuck during more detailed questioning. In any event, to have been involved in innovatory work is good enough experience in itself and is worth mentioning.

2 You can work with other professionals and probably have good interpersonal skills.

3 You carry things through (*'While progress was initially slow...'*) and persevere towards your goal. If you cite very recent experience, be prepared to be questioned about evidence of success.

4 You are concerned with the patients' quality of life. Gaining or regaining social skills is crucially important to these patients, especially if they are to rejoin the community.

5 You are a problem solver. You have not only recognised the problem that most institutionalised patients tend to communicate through their carers rather than directly with each other, but you have taken steps to solve the problem.

6 You can work alone. The speech therapist is 'visiting' and therefore not present at all of your daily group meetings.

7 You can supervise and teach other members of staff. You are not on duty all the time, so clearly other nurses on the ward have learned how to lead the group towards its goal.

8 You have organisational skills.

There is, in fact, quite a lot to be read into this short paragraph which would not be obvious from the description of the current post held on the application form or CV. It is clear that you have the necessary experience for the grade G post, and other skills besides.

THE ACCOMPANYING LETTER

You should include with your application form or CV a short covering letter, handwritten or typed, on plain writing paper – not hospital writing paper (which might be seen as stealing) nor a sheet torn from a notebook. Your letter should refer to the job advertisement, to your visit or telephone call, if you made one (unless you made a hash of it, in which case it is better not to draw attention to your mistake), and give just one good reason why you should be considered for the job. Figure 5.2 gives an example of such a letter.

Mr T Sebastian
Lindsell Hospital
Walden, Northants
May 19, 1989

Dear Mr Sebastian

I should like to apply for the post of sister in the intensive care unit of Lindsell Hospital, advertised in *Nursing Times*, May 17, 1989.

I have been in my present post as senior staff nurse in the ICU at Adams Hospital for just over a year, and I have gained confidence and experience in the specialty. I should now like to put that experience to use in a more responsible position.

I was particularly interested in the research project currently taking place in the Lindsell ICU and would very much like to participate in it.

I enclose my application form and look forward to hearing from you.

Yours sincerely,

Claire Vickers

Figure 5.2   *The accompanying letter*

Before you post it

Read through what you have written, just in case any mistakes have slipped in. Take a copy of everything, so you have something to refer to when you are called for interview.

Figure 5.3 summarises the steps involved in completing an application form or CV.

FURTHER READING

Skeats, Judy, *CVs and Written Applications* (Ward Lock, 1987).

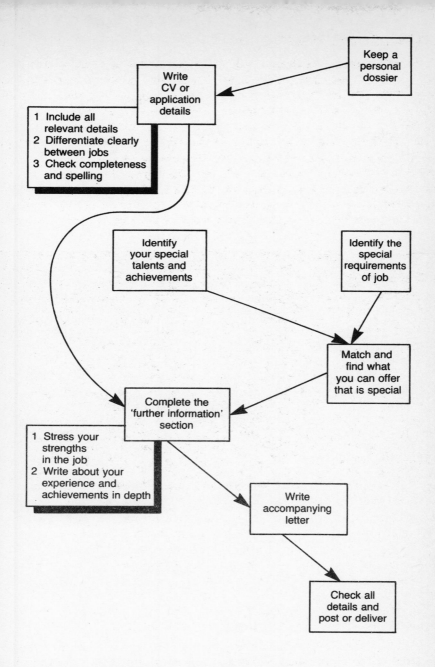

Figure 5.3 *Application form and CV summary chart*

Chapter 6

THE CANDIDATE SELECTION PROCESS OVERALL

OVERVIEW OF RECRUITMENT STAGES

A full account of good practice from the selectors' point of view is given in Chapter 18. This chapter gives a summary of the likely process the candidate has to face. Flowchart A, on page 2, shows the process from the candidate's perspective while flowchart B, on page 113, shows it from that of the employer.

For the employer, selection should start with a review. This involves taking stock of whether the vacancy needs to be filled, whether the job should be changed, and what kind of person should be sought to fill it. Quite often no review takes place. The advertisement is placed without time being wasted on any such introspection. There may not have been any thought given to the requirements from candidates.

When the advertisement is placed, a plan should exist that lays out all of the stages in recruitment, usually in this order:

- Placing of advertisements.
- Closing date for applications.
- Acknowledgement of applications.
- Shortlisting meeting.
- Invitations to attend for interview.
- Regret letters to unshortlisted candidates.
- Arrangements for informal visits.
- Interview dates.
- Dates of other assessments.
- Taking up of references (could be before the interview).
- Medical checks.

- Offer of post(s) to successful candidate(s).
- Advice and/or letters of 'regret' to unsuccessful candidates.

Let us now look at these stages in relation to the candidate. Since Chapters 3 and 4 have covered advertisements and informal visits from the candidate's point of view, they will not be discussed further here.

CLOSING DATE FOR APPLICATIONS

It is surprising how often advertisements appear that give only a day or two for reply. Normally, two or three weeks should be allowed. You may see the advertisement late, if you do not get the *Nursing Times* passed to you until others have seen it. It is sometimes worth ringing the advertiser's personnel department and asking if they will extend the closing date, on the grounds that you have just seen the advertisement and it would appear to be a post for which you are well suited and would like to apply for.

SHORTLISTING MEETING

Normally, the interview panel meets within a week of the closing date to decide who to shortlist.

Shortlisting is a screening process that allows candidates who appear less suitable on paper to be dropped. Sometimes this is done through a careful analysis of application forms, assessing candidates against criteria using relevant information. More often, however, it is done more subjectively, in terms of people saying 'This one looks quite good, let's see her', or by making inferences from handwriting about character, or from job history about past success. Quite often the objective is simply to keep the number of 'seen' candidates down to manageable numbers, and the judges may be hard put to explain why some candidates were preferred over others.

In the past, the ritual of shortlisting has remained secret. Nowadays, like all other interview processes, it may be tested in an industrial tribunal for its fairness. In theory, shortlisting panels would then have to produce evidence of how they carried out the task fairly, and be able to show that they consistently applied criteria that were not unfairly discriminatory. In practice, it is hard for people aggrieved at not being shortlisted to find out how such decisions were made, unless they have some independent evidence of unfair discrimination to begin with.

Shortlisting decisions are made almost entirely (for outside candidates) on the strength of what candidates put in writing. Few people will be rejected at this stage because they are *over*-qualified. If you are not shortlisted, but expected to be, you might want to ask why. You are almost bound to get a bland response, such as 'Well, we had a lot of very good candidates, and some of them had more relevant experience/qualifications than you.'

INVITATIONS TO THE INTERVIEW

You should normally expect to receive this about a week after the closing date and a week or two before the interview. Two weeks before is reasonable, as people need to arrange to have the time off, but sometimes employers call people in with only a day or two's notice. What will this say to you about their consideration for employees' interests?

Sometimes employers will indicate that if you do not hear from them within two weeks of the closing date, you can assume that your application has not been successful, thus dispensing with the costs and courtesies of acknowledgement and personal letters of regret.

INTERVIEW DATES

These are normally within three weeks of the closing date. Rarely are candidates given a choice, but frequently there is some flexibility possible, if you are shortlisted and they are keen to have a look at you. Do try to rearrange it if you are ill. You may find that the time you are given is a problem. It will invariably be possible to change to a different time on the same day.

DATES OF OTHER ASSESSMENTS

The interview is normally the last event in the assessment process. Any other assessments normally take place on the interview day, although sometimes they happen a few days before – often the day before. Chapter 10 gives advice on handling these.

TAKING UP OF REFERENCES

You will probably be asked for the names of referees on the application form. You may be asked to indicate whether referees can be contacted immediately, when you are shortlisted, or only if you are offered the post. If you say only if offered the post, you may arouse a little suspicion. On the other hand, you would not want your referees contacted prematurely. I recommend that you say that you would want them contacted only if you are shortlisted. Rarely do employers take up references on all applications. Sometimes in the health service they are only taken up after the interview.

You will need to select your referees with care. They should meet the following criteria:

- They should know you personally.
- They should know your work.
- They could be credible judges of your suitability for the post for which you have applied.
- They should have some professional status.
- They will give you a reasonable reference.
- Preferably, they will show you or tell you what they have written.
- One should be your current supervising officer.

Don't forget to ask them first.

MEDICAL CHECKS

These are carried out around the time of the interview. All the interviewers should be told by their occupational health department whether or not there is any health impediment to you doing a job, assuming they offer you one. Your medical details remain confidential.

OFFER OF POST(S) TO SUCCESSFUL CANDIDATE(S)

You will normally know a day or two after the interview. This is covered later in Chapter 13.

LETTERS OF 'REGRET' TO UNSUCCESSFUL CANDIDATES

These are fairly standard and tell you nothing of course. If you want to know why you didn't get the job, you will have to ask nicely. This is covered in Chapter 13.

Chapter 7

ALL ABOUT THE INTERVIEW

When going for an interview, your objective must be to be offered the job that you want. So you must be sure of what you want. You must be able to find out sufficient information to know that this job is the right one for you. You must ensure that you will come across well enough to be offered it.

WHAT YOU ARE IN FOR

You will have already made some judgements based on the kind of reception your initial enquiry received on the telephone, on the style of the letter inviting you to interview, and perhaps on the willingness of people to take you around the workplace before the interview. If you are left hanging on the telephone, if your application cannot be found, or if, before the interview, everyone seems too busy for courtesies or to take an interest in your particular needs and questions, then you may well feel that they are not worth bothering with at all. Sadly, this is all too often the case.

At best, an interview is an open and friendly affair, where you will have ample opportunity to get to know the people and observe them behaving quite naturally – and also build up some confidence that the judgements of the people you meet will be fair.

A poor interview could be very different. It could be described as a stilted ritual carried out under stress, producing a quite untypical sample of the candidate's behaviour, from which quite unjustified conclusions are drawn on the basis of the inter-viewer's prejudices.

THEIR OBJECTIVES

Interviewers usually see their role as filling a vacancy or finding a replacement for someone who has left. Emphasis is on finding someone who is competent and able to 'fit in', and the application form, references and interview are seen as the only means of doing this.

Good, experienced interviewers will have a clear idea of what they are looking for. This will be expressed in terms of criteria. They will be seeking definite evidence that you meet the criteria they have set. If you have been sent a list of requirements that the successful candidate must possess, then this is a sign that the interview is going to be quite systematic and that the interviewers have some expertise in assessment.

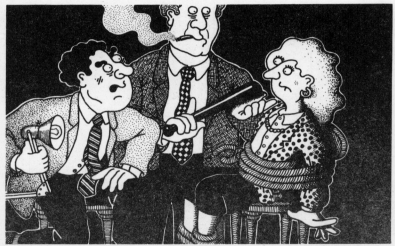

The possession of a list of requirements (often called the 'person specification') will help you in deciding whether to apply. It is sometimes sent to you with the information pack, and occasionally with an interview briefing. More often than not, you do not get it, and have to infer what the employer wants from publicity about the job. If you have this list, it might suggest an open approach on their part (and vice versa). It will not tell you *how* they intend to go about assessing you.

At the end of the interviews, the selectors want to be able to make two kinds of decision:

1 Who meets the criteria and who does not.
2 Who is the best of those who do.

INTERVIEW JUDGEMENTS

Although the interview is the favoured method for selection, it is not a particularly accurate way of finding out about people. Sometimes the judgements made are poor predictors of subsequent performance.

In order to do better than chance, interviewers must be clear about what they are looking for and be trained to elicit concrete evidence to back up their judgements, rather than simply rely on impressions.

There are good reasons why interviews are not very good at getting to the truth about people. Interviewers very rarely get any feedback on their work. It is like having to diagnose and treat a problem without any knowledge of outcomes. True, interviewers sometimes have to live with their failures, but there is no way of telling whether the adverse judgements of those who are not subsequently employed are sound or not. Neither is it common to seek detailed follow-up of the truth of the judgements of those selected.

You might like to read Chapter 24 to find out what kinds of errors of judgement are made by interviewers. It is the notion of being judged that candidates find inhibiting, of course, and the power that interviewers have inevitably leads to a less than truthful self-presentation by candidates. Candidates are also often judged on how well they talk about their performance, rather than on how well they actually perform it.

THEY WILL BE IN CONTROL

The interviewers are in control but there is a pretence of normal social contact. The better you can relate (or achieve 'rapport'), the more positively you are likely to be judged. If you feel relaxed and prepared to trust the interviewers as people, you are more likely to want to come over as yourself, rather than put on an act for the interview. They will control the length of the interview, but you can control the number of questions asked by the length of your answers.

FIRST IMPRESSIONS COUNT

As substantial judgements about candidates are often made in the first four minutes, your initial presentation is going to be vital.

Interview conventions require you to be friendly (even if some interviewers purposely make a point of being distinctly unfriendly); to be prepared to sell yourself, by telling the truth (but embellishing it slightly is allowable, and even expected). Some of the questions will be straightforward; others will be tricky. You will be expected to read the coded messages and give the interviewers what they want, or be found wanting yourself. You, not they, will be blamed for any failure in communication that occurs.

Many interviewers see their jobs as simply one of judging, as if they were at a dog show. Often, much less attention is given to the needs and worries of potential candidates. Interviewers are less aware than they should be of the candidate's right to *judge them*.

All too often, little effort is made to present the organisation as friendly and welcoming and one worth working for. Yet interviews have a considerable meaning in terms of public relations.

THE COMMON PATTERN

If you analyse the typical interview, you will find a common pattern: formal greeting; some chit-chat to relax everyone; a statement of what it is about; questions on home background, education and training, and clinical interests, why you want the job and what you think you can offer, your future aspirations; the terms and conditions; a chance for you to ask questions; details about the decision and further contact; thanks and goodbyes.

A typical interviewer checklist will include a note to find out about:

- personality
- attitude to patients and to authority
- ability to work on your own
- ability to assume responsibility
- concern for safety
- clinical competence and judgement
- clinical interests
- ability to work with and/or supervise others
- ability to communicate.

Standards are rarely written down – they are in the interviewers' minds. Many will not have a clear plan for getting this information when they start the interview.

It is a formidable task to get reliable evidence on all of these things in 20 minutes or so. You will be seeking to remove any doubts they may have about you.

Being successful in selling yourself will depend partly on giving the right impression. It will also depend on your ability to co-operate and communicate with the interviewers in their quest for positive evidence about you.

At the same time, you will want to eliminate all damaging negative impressions. Interviewers, on the other hand, will be trying to find ways (sometimes devious) of digging for negative aspects. Many interviewers attach a lot of weight to the discovery of anything detrimental (like the hint of a bad relationship with someone). They may have been trained to probe it relentlessly. But you must decide whether presenting yourself as perfect may be restricting for you. In the long run, it might be better to be honest. They may not believe that you are perfect, even if you are!

WHAT IS THE EMPLOYER LOOKING FOR?

You are indeed fortunate if your information pack has given you a detailed person specification to study and work on. Naturally, each job will have its own demands, and each panel will have its own ideas of important aspects. It will be helpful if we look at the interviewer's checklist again now, with a view to identifying more closely what may be critical in the context of a particular job. We shall call this a person specification for a clinical job. In Chapter 10, we will look at personnel specifications for other kinds of jobs, including managerial ones.

Person specification – basic clinical post

This might apply, for instance, to a senior staff nurse (E) or ward sister's (G) post. The requirements marked '*' are ones where experience is a factor – that is, your ability increases with practice.

Personality and motivation

Rarely is a certain type of personality specified. 'Well motivated' is everywhere. People with energy, and who are conscientious

61

and stable, are in demand. People who do not panic in a crisis, and who are naturally cheerful and open, are useful people to have around. The interviewer will be looking for defects rather than strengths or any one type of profile.

Attitude to patients and to authority

Most employers would be keen to detect any hint of a rejecting or unco-operative attitude here. Perhaps too much deference or timidity might be a problem.

Ability to work on one's own

This is related partly to the ability to function without support (that is, to be psychologically autonomous), rather than dependent, and also to be capable of doing things without constant guidance – perhaps related to general competence in such a situation.

Ability to assume responsibility*

Most professional jobs require people to take charge and make decisions when a boss is absent. Also, to 'take the can back' for one's own actions.

Concern for safety*

This is a fairly obvious requirement. Again, this might be reflected partly by personality and partly by training.

Clinical competence and judgement*

This will need closer definition in the context that is required. The statutory competencies and NHS clinical grading definitions are important, defining the major competencies for which people receive specified grades.

Clinical interests shown

This is not the same as competence at all. It may be important in showing a person's general commitment to nursing; how keen she is in keeping up to date; and whether any special interests are likely to be of use in a particular job – or even frustrated in a particular job. Also, does she have a sufficient interest to do some spare time reading?

Ability to work with and/or supervise others*

This means both mixing well with others and being able to lead. How adaptable is the individual towards people? Does she always want to be 'one of the girls', afraid to be unpopular when her responsibilities demand it?

Ability to communicate*

This can mean a whole host of things. It could be taken to mean the ability of the person to say clearly what she means, whether in reports or in conversation. However, it might mean influencing other people to her own views.

FURTHER READING

Fletcher, Clive, *How to Face the Interview*, 2nd Edn (Unwin, 1988).

Chapter 8

HONEST SELF-APPRAISAL

Genius does what it must and talent does what it can.

Owen Meredith

You must first identify the requirements of the job. If it is a clinical post, you must study the job description and the person specification, if you have one. Many of the requirements that employers seek are described in Chapter 16.

Use your findings to make headings, as specific as you can, for what you believe the employer requires. You must use this to test your own suitability. You must do this with total honesty – you are the client in this appraisal.

FIRST STAGE: HOW DO YOU COMPARE?

Using the specification you have drawn up, try to get some idea of where you stand when you compare yourself with each of those requirements. On each point, rate yourself somewhere on the following scale:

1 Excellent – this is one of my major strengths.
2 I am generally good, but could possibly improve.
3 No more than adequate.
4 Definitely weak – I could improve with practice and training.
5 Hopeless – a definite 'blind spot'.

Note your shortfalls and decide what to do about them.

Do not be afraid of asking others their opinion of you, if you feel you can. Nurses often have a poor opinion of themselves, or set standards for themselves that are too high.

SECOND STAGE: ASSESSING SCOPE FOR DEVELOPMENT IN THE JOB

Decide how critical your weaknesses might be in that particular job. For instance, if your weakness is in a certain clinical area, is it possible that the employer would allow you to develop your knowledge and skills while in the post?

THIRD STAGE: DECIDING IF YOU ARE A VIABLE CANDIDATE

Do you still want to try for the post? The results of your analysis may be that you are so far short of the requirements that you would have little chance of success. Or possibly that if the employer was misguided enough to take you on, you would find it impossible to live up to the expectations. Trying to do so might be very painful for you.

FOURTH STAGE: IDENTIFYING YOUR STRATEGY

We assume now that you still want to go ahead with your application for a particular job. In this application, and in the interview, you will be trying to make the most of your strengths. This is covered in the next chapter.

As far as your weaknesses are concerned, you need first of all to ask 'Are they in important areas as far as this job is concerned?' You may then do a number of things.

Be honest

Admit weaknesses (as development needs), without being too self-effacing, and make your determination to develop apparent. If the interview is an open two-way process, like an appraisal, then this may be useful. You put yourself in the hands of the interviewers, and rely on their goodwill. If the failing is something that you feel you should have overcome by now, you may be embarrassed to admit it. You are on safer ground here in jobs that are clearly ones where training is offered.

Adopt the salesman's approach – 'we hope you won't ask'

Conceal them, by not bringing attention to them in your CV or in the interview. You hope they will not ask or probe too deeply. The skilled candidate hopes to have sufficient control in the interview to be able to deflect probing questions.

Tell a white lie

This is the risky tactic. You may be found out – through references, for instance, or even by determined probing on the part of the interviewer. You may sell yourself into the wrong job, by concealing your weaknesses.

SKELETONS IN THE CUPBOARD

In reviewing your suitability, you may well be all too painfully aware of something that is likely to put you at a considerable disadvantage, like a chronic health problem or disability, or a 'black mark' against you because you have a poor work record or have been in some sort of trouble with authority. Let us look at these problems separately.

Health problems

Strictly speaking, it is not up to the interviewers to investigate a health problem. They should, in theory, judge your suitability on other grounds, leaving it to the occupational health department to tell them whether they recommend you for employment in the post. If you are too ill to attend the interview, or have had considerable time off work recently (which will come out in the references), you need to consider your application carefully. You may well have to resign yourself to missing the opportunity, unless you have a good advocate, or the employer is prepared to wait.

The poor record

If you have had a lot of time off work in the past, you must be prepared to provide evidence that this will not re-occur. If you suffer from recurrent problems, you might still be considered, but you would need to provide reassurances, and possibly seek a more flexible contract – to work part-time, or as a locum, or through an agency (you might set up your own). If you have a disability, there may be inducements to the employer to employ you – most will seek to improve their record of employing disabled people if they can be convinced that the disability will not impede your effectiveness.

A poor performance record must be explained as well. Perhaps you were in the wrong job and are seeking a chance to turn over a new leaf and prove yourself in your new job. Most people will probably be unprepared to confess to a poor work record, but the referee might refer to it, with or without any mitigating circumstances you may mention at the interview.

The disciplinary record

You may have been through a bad patch with your current employer, as a result of which you have found yourself with a formal disciplinary warning on your file. If it is current, you need to make sure that your reference will not blight your chances. Your boss, as a referee, will probably have to refer to it, however obliquely. Your best chance will be to plead that the trouble is behind you, and that you have made amends and learned your lesson. A good referee can support this. You should also maintain that, given a fresh start, you will be in no danger of relapsing.

Criminal convictions

Health services employment is generally exempted from the Rehabilitation of Offenders Act where, after a certain period free from re-occurrence, convictions are seen as 'spent' and cannot be referred to.

If you decide not to declare any criminal conviction you may have, even if 'spent', you may be faced with dismissal if the truth leaks out later. It is recommended that you explain the circumstances and plead that the trouble is behind you, and at the same time make sure that you have two good referees who can vouch for your current integrity.

Figure 8.1 summarises the steps involved in honest self-appraisal.

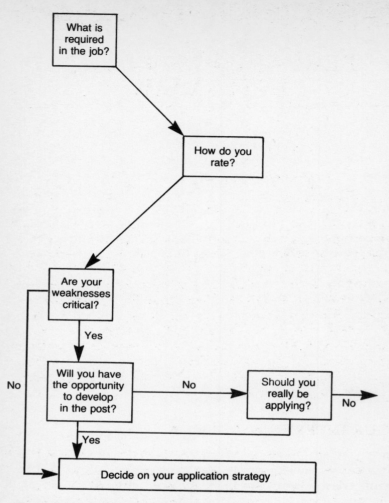

Figure 8.1 *Self-appraisal summary chart*

REFERENCE

HMSO, *Rehabilitation of Offenders Act* (HMSO, 1974).

FURTHER READING

Tschudin, Verena, *Managing Yourself*, Essentials of Nursing Management series (Macmillan, 1990).

Chapter 9

PREPARING FOR THE INTERVIEW

As for disappointing them, I should not so much mind; but I can't abide
to disappoint myself.   Oliver Goldsmith, *She Stoops to Conquer*

You need to ensure that the interview arrangements will give
you time to find out all that you need to and to prepare yourself
properly. Some employers always seem to be in a frantic rush to
get candidates to interviews, and will not allow time for the
informal visit or for the consideration of candidates' questions
and concerns prior to the interview. Unless you are desperate
yourself, you will be wise to be wary of the desperate, poorly
organised, or inconsiderate employer.

YOUR INTERVIEW AGENDA

Once you are asked to attend for interview, you need to
consider how you are going to put across your strengths during
the interview. Do not assume that the interviewers will necessarily have read (or remembered) what you have said about
yourself. You will need to have an agenda of your strong points,
and be sure you can respond to opportunities to present them.

Remember that you have to decide whether you want to
admit to your weaknesses or play them down. (If you lie
outright, you are likely to come unstuck if they start probing
you.) If you are open about weaknesses, you may prevent
yourself being offered a job that would be unsuitable, and in
which you may well be unhappy or unsuccessful. If may be best
to check out beforehand whether a certain deficiency would be a
handicap.

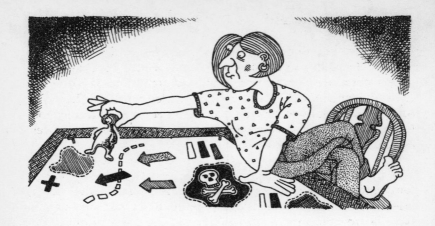

Openness about your faults may well suggest that you are a self-aware and honest person. Perhaps you are admitting to a lack of experience that would be expected in your situation, and which could be easily remedied. On the other hand, you may be hoping that they will not ask you about some things, but you need to have an answer ready in case they do ask questions. They may get information on any of these areas from references, but they will not want to take the referees' word for it.

THE INTERVIEWERS' CUES

Appearances and body language

Firstly, interviewers go on *appearances*, or here and now impressions. Here, the body language clues you give are as important as what you say. You must aim to come across as friendly and confident (but not over-confident), and walk into the room with an upright posture. Cringing and avoiding eye contact, which are natural responses of a nervous person, may be read as indicating a shifty nature. Folded arms may suggest defensiveness; covering the mouth, dishonesty. So be aware of how you appear when nervous, and work hard to overcome your mannerisms. Above all, work at staying relaxed. This is not easy, but if you are petrified and shaking like a jelly, you are not going to be able to do well or give any impression of confidence. If you are able to say that you feel nervous to the interviewers, they are often able to respond sympathetically, and that helps.

70

Exploring your record

In going about their task, some interviewers will have the benefit of training and some not: some will be confident and others nervous. Hence, there will be a great deal of scope for their idiosyncracies, pet questions and clever tricks. They will draw you into unwelcome areas and get you to say things you had not intended to. There will be some embarrassing silences and some misunderstandings.

One standard opening gambit is to ask you to explain why you are applying for the job. What answer should you give? A fairly modest response is effective. If you have some career interests, mention the job as a career step; if not, stress what you have heard about the sound practice at the place in question. Interviewers like to think that their job is special and want to hear that you value their institution. If you say what they want to hear, they are likely to judge you as well-motivated. If you are more honest and say 'Well, it's a job. . .', they will assume that you have not given it much thought, or that you are a drifter who does not act purposefully.

Many interviews start with 'Let us go through your career to date. . .' or 'Why did you take up nursing?'. They may ask you to talk about your education, giving examples of your favourite subjects or work areas. These are normally safe starting points. They also give you the chance to show your self-confidence and ability to relate to people.

Alternatively, they may start with the here and now, why you want a change, how you came to be where you are, and so on to a series of confusing 'and before that. . .' questions.

They will be probing what you have done in the past, and will come to some conclusions about your competence on the basis of your answers. In your application form or CV, the facts will speak for themselves, but they will want to go further in the interview. They are seeking facts about what you have done, as well as how and why you have done it. The answers might give them clues as to your motivation and personality. The record is a basis for probing beneath the surface, into what you did not say.

Interviewers tend to search out negative evidence and can ignore the positive. Here, you can prepare by getting a friend to quiz you, to make sure that you can come over without hesitation or mumbling. The friend should probe you, asking why and how, as well as what.

Hypothetical and test questions

Interviewers may rely on hypothetical or test questions which start 'If you were... how would you?'. You are not likely to be able to guess the pet questions (unless you have a friend who has been through it beforehand – this is always worth checking). However, learning to respond on the spot to hypothetical questions can be improved by practice.

Hypothetical questions may be difficult if they relate to unfamiliar circumstances. Check whether these questions are inviting you to mention a number of issues, or whether they want you to give one specific answer. It is often safer to answer more generally and mention different aspects. Do not be afraid to ask for clarification or to check that you are giving the kind of answer they want.

Any claim of clinical knowledge that you make is liable to be tested. If you say you are well up on the latest research, do have something to quote!

The interviewers are trying to ascertain whether you meet their standards in these areas. A good interviewer will be probing to find out, from the work you have done, whether you are able to maintain your standards under pressure, and what tricky situations you have had to handle that have tested these qualities. Make sure you give clear and complete answers to these questions. When they say 'Was there anything else?', take it as a clue to refer to some other aspect you haven't yet mentioned.

Occasionally, you will be given a series of test questions to do on paper. These may be separate from the interview.

They will be observing how you express yourself

Your communication skill is often assessed by how well you come across under the stress of an interview. This is not really fair, but you will need to make sure that you can stay relaxed before and during the interview in order to be at your best. You may find relaxation exercises useful. Alternatively, you may like to bring some reading to occupy you during the inevitable periods of waiting.

They listen for a hint of problems with people

It is here that some interviewers will behave like amateur social workers, trying to gauge from your background whether you have had stability and a sound family environment. Some of their questions will be simply inviting you to talk about your relationships at work and at home.

PREPARATION STAGE BY STAGE

Your interview preparation should include the items listed in the following checklist.

Checklist 9.1

1 Your list of their requirements.
2 The list of your strengths and weaknesses (Chapter 8), from which you identify selling points and weak points.
3 A list of questions to which you need to have previously thought out answers.
4 A study of what you said on your CV and/or application form.
5 Your own questions about the job.
6 A rehearsal with a friend who simulates the questions and gives you feedback on how you come across, verbally and non-verbally. The friend should also prepare some relevant test questions about clinical (or managerial) practice and current events.
7 A timetable and checklist of what you need to do on the day to ensure you get to the interview in plenty of time, relaxed and confidently prepared.
8 A good night's sleep the night before.

Your list of their requirements

If you have not done this yet, work through the suggested procedure in Chapter 8.

Selling points

Your self-appraisal in Chapters 5 and 8 will have brought out your strengths and weaknesses in relation to the job. Now is the time to make a list of the strong points:

I am suitable for this job because. . .

I will have no problem with. . . because. . .

You need to be able to back up each statement of a strength with examples:

because. . .

. . .I have often had to. . .

. . .that is something I enjoy. . .

. . .people have told me I am good at this. . .

. . .in six years I have never had that problem. . .

. . .I get lots of practice in this. . .

Here is an example of what might be said:

I know I will be able to handle the paperwork on the wards because I have frequently acted as sister and had to take responsibility for that.

Weak points

Remember that we said in Chapter 8 that you had to decide whether to admit or conceal these.

Admission

This may involve saying:

I admit that I do not have that experience. . .

I admit that I am not very good at that. . .

. . .but I am very keen to learn about it. . .

. . .but I have studied it in books. . .

. . .but I am actively working on it. . .

. . .but I have made some considerable improvements in this. . .

. . .but I have done such and such which is quite similar. . .

. . .but it has not been necessary/much of a problem to date. . .

Or:

I have made mistakes in the past. . .

. . .but that is behind me now. . .

. . .but I learned a lot from it. . .

Concealment

If they touch on your Achilles heel, you will need to rehearse saying something like:

I cannot tell you about that but you may be interested in. . .

That is, something else that might sound rather similar. Or you will hope that they won't ask, and it is amazing how often they do not!

Questions you need to have answers to

The following example gives some standard questions, together with an indication of what the interviewer is usually seeking by asking it, and some hints about how you should answer.

Example

Questions and what they are getting at	Hints on how to respond
1 Competence: *What can this person do?*	You must go for positive responses.
Are you able to. . .? Have you ever. . .?	Straightforward, direct questions. If the answer is no, you might say 'No, but I can do. . .'
What are your strengths. . . and weaknesses?	Difficult to think this one out on your feet. Strengths should be job-related ones and weaknesses should be irrelevant to the job.
How would you cope with. . .?	A leading question – answer 'no problem' but explain why.
How would you do such and such?	Testing your knowledge, as in a clinical assessment.
Sell me this (or this idea). . .	A pet question, usually on a pet subject – some version of the nursing process or clinical procedure. They may want to see how persuasive you are.

---

2   Previous and current jobs:
    Where has this person been?
    What has she gained?
    Is there a pattern?
    Does she know what she wants?
    What did it involve?

    It is worth going right through your CV with all of these questions.

    What did you like best... and least... about it?

    Why did you leave?
    How has your career to date prepared you for this job?

    Similar questions are often asked about training.

3   Motives:
    Will this person stick at it?
    Are her interests deep enough?
    Is she career motivated?

    Why did you apply for this job?
    Why do you want to work here?
    What do you really enjoy in the work?
    Where have you most enjoyed working?

    You will be wise to have answers that relate to the job on offer.

    Where do you see yourself in three years' time.

    You have to be ambitious, but don't overdo it, or they will think you pushy or likely to push off quickly.

    Tell me about your career to date...

    Be ready to summarise in a few words. Give positive highlights.

4   Personality:
    Will she fit in?
    Lead others?
    Be stable?

    Tell me something about yourself...

    A horrible question. It may just be a rather bad starter question.

    What are your interests outside work?

    Stress job-related skills.

What makes you angry?

Be as honest as you want to be, but avoid sounding unreasonable, weird, insensitive, over-confident, petty or mean.

How would others describe you?

5 Awareness:
Does she know what's going on?
Understand the world and herself?

What was the last book/ clinical article you read?
Do you know about...
(something topical)?

This is just to warn you that you should be prepared for a few topical 'hot potatoes', especially professional talking points.

What are your strengths...
and weaknesses?
How would others describe you?

These questions are also assessing self-awareness.

6 Circumstances:
Is this person prepared to make herself sufficiently available?

Do you know where you would live?
Are you mobile?
Could you work irregular hours?

These questions often seem prying. They may only be checking on how much you've thought about the changes you would have to make, or simply checking your availability for unexpected overtime. Some may be devious ways of checking the strength of your domestic commitments.

How would you manage to look after your children?
Are you thinking of starting a family?

These are clearly discriminatory questions. Do not show anger. You need not answer. Try asking politely why the question has been asked.

Study of your CV and application form

We do sometimes get carried away on paper, and it can be embarrassing to be reminded of it at the interview. So check that you are aware and can back up everything you say. If you say you like reading clinical research papers, try to have one to quote.

Your own questions about the job

These are likely to be of two types:

1   Questions that you really want to know the answers to.
2   Questions that might impress the panel.

The first are based on the list of things that you have made out as your own requirements. It is fine to ask questions about practice and facilities, but it is not advisable to ask about additional 'perks' they might offer you in the interview itself – you might seem mercenary if you do. Some of your queries could be directed to the personnel staff.

Questions to impress usually start with 'I was very interested to note that. . .' or 'I have a special interest in. . . would there be scope in this post for. . .?'.

Remember that interviewers are generally behind time, and so they do not appreciate candidates who bring out a list of 15 penetrating questions from their briefcase or handbag. Do not spoil your good impression by making them yawn or feel irritable.

Rehearsal

Learning a set script is not going to help you. You probably won't get the chance to use it, and if you do, you will not sound natural.

The best approach is to go through some simulated interview questions the evening before with a friend pretending to be the interviewer. She should note how well you reply – perhaps you might record the conversation. You will also want to know how well your 'selling points' come over, and how you coped with questions about weak areas.

It will certainly be useful to make a list of questions you want to ask and of points you want to make sure you make in promotion of your case.

Interviews will always be unpredictable, and the judgements of people will always be subject to bias and impressions. However, if you prepare sensibly, anticipating some of the issues, you are likely to put yourself over better.

Do not forget at the end of the day that you are also making a decision, and that the interviewers and the organisation they represent must come up to your standards as a professional employee.

TYPES OF INTERVIEW

There are various types of interview depending on the job, organisation and interviewers. These are summarised in Table 9.1. (See Chapter 17 for a discussion of selection options, from the interviewer's point of view.)

Table 9.1   *Types of interview*

Types of interview	Characterised by	Likely problems for candidates
Formal	Ritual introductions; evident chairperson; formal introductions and turns for interviewers; clear structure; restrained manner; sombre setting; large table	Staying relaxed; understanding the etiquette
Informal	Friendly, relaxed setting; little formality; possibly free structure; often no table	Being caught off guard; false *bonhomie*; sometimes too unstructured and open ended
Sequential	A series of interviews (usually two) conducted by different people; success in one may confer entry to the other (a screening process), or all candidates may have to undergo all of them	Being clear what each is for and which matters most; repetition of questions
Competitive	Typically one job and several candidates	Additional stress of rivalry

Table 9.1 (*cont.*)

Types of interview	Characterised by	Likely problems for candidates
Screening	All who reach a set standard will be taken on	Estimating the standard
Stress	The interview is an ordeal testing the 'mettle' of candidates	Staying cool; rapport; deciding whether you want to join

FURTHER READING

Fletcher, Clive, *A Guide to Self Preparation and Presentation* (Unwin Press, 1981).

Higham, Martin, *Coping with Interviews*, Revised Edn (New Opportunity Press, 1983).

Mackenzie, Davey, D and McDonnel, P, *How to Be Interviewed* (British Institute of Management, 1980).

Silverman, M A, 'How to lose a job', *Management Today*, September 1978.

Yate, Martin, J, *Great Answers to Tough Interview Questions: How to Get the Job You Want*, 2nd Edn (Kogan Page, 1988).

Chapter 10

SELECTION FOR SENIOR AND MANAGERIAL POSTS

It is not enough to succeed – others must fail.

Gore Vidal

If you are going for a management job, or a very senior position, you are likely to be subjected to a more elaborate selection procedure. In this chapter, we look at some of the things that you may have to face.

The more elaborate procedure is likely to involve more people, more events, more criteria and more organisational ritual. By organisational ritual, I mean events that are seen as socially necessary but which often add little to the quality of assessment. Let us take a look at these first.

ORGANISATIONAL RITUAL

Where a manager who will be taking decisions affecting a number of people is appointed, there is a need to demonstrate to people who are powerful in the organisation, like senior medical staff and managers, that the process is being done openly, and that the powerful people are offered some token involvement. It is a chance for senior management to see who might be joining, and to have their say if there is some candidate they vehemently object to.

Similarly, candidates considered important enough are given the opportunity to meet senior people in an informal setting, and (in theory) to ask them pertinent questions. Since this is done as part of the selection procedure, but superficially and unsystematically, the assessments by either side of the other's qualities are likely to be very impressionistic. It is not unheard of for a candidate to withdraw on the basis of what she discovered at some informal gathering during selection. For most people, it is an ordeal, a rite of passage to be managed as best you can.

THE TRIAL-BY-SHERRY PARTY

It is 6 p.m. in the Committee Room at the district headquarters. Tomorrow there will be interviews for a senior post in the district.

Half an hour ago the caterers added the finishing touches to a lavish buffet. A secretary is distributing copies of potted biographies of the candidates. Name badges are being issued, and the wine is being uncorked.

Twenty minutes later, the 'trial by sherry' is in full swing. An invitation by the district general manager is an invitation to participate by making searching observations and asking probing questions of the candidates.

The current differences between district directors are forgotten in a display of *bonhomie* and wit. The room is noisy with chatter. There are 25 people present, with district officers clustered in groups of three or four around the candidates. Afterwards, some of the officers will be invited to a private meeting with the district general manager, to give their impressions. Maybe they will say that they liked Mrs A, who had enthusiasm and interesting ideas. They did not go for Mr B who seemed pompous and lacked any discernible sense of humour. Mr C was a bit of a non-entity, unlike Mr D who was rather overwhelming and had had too much to drink. Miss E was so nervous that no one could get much out of her, and the man from the Department of Social Security, Mr F, was a bit of an oddball. Mr G was young and naïve, and they could not see him handling the unit general managers and the rather overbearing deputy that he would have to work with.

It certainly takes experience to deal with this kind of event, and extroverts have an advantage – you will need to have learned to balance your wine glass in one hand, the paper plate and serviette in the other, and to avoid choking on a slice of quiche or spilling the wine over the district general manager when he asks your views on resource management.

You will need to have practised the art of saying nothing very much, while sounding intelligent, and of withholding an opinion until you are sure of the views of your interrogator. You will know that you need to make some kind of impact, but it must be a positive one, so you will drink only orange juice. You will also force yourself to listen very carefully to the questions, trying to pick up any clues about your interrogator's prejudices and enthusiasms. But you will avoid getting into conversations that are out of your depth.

You will have learned that it is wise to find out as much as you can about the authority before you attend such an event, so you can ask intelligent questions – asking questions is a good tactic because it helps to take the pressure off of you.

These gatherings are far worse for most candidates than the organisers ever imagine. The latter see them as pleasant and natural social gatherings, where everyone can talk in a relaxed and informal way, and be themselves in a way that is not possible at the interview. Certainly, the candidate who collapsed when rising from her chair because her legs had gone numb with fear did not feel this way.

The consolation might be that such events are fairly token affairs, and provided you do nothing too bizarre, they are unlikely to be the reason for your disqualification from consideration. On the other hand, they provide useful opportunities for you to see the people you might be working with, at play, and to pick up some useful signals about their morale and their styles. You may or may not see them as a group of people with whom you will be able to relate as colleagues.

PRELIMINARY WORK

For some management posts, you are asked to write an essay or a report, giving your views. One suspects that sometimes this is a way of getting some free management consultancy from the candidates, or at least picking their brains for some new ideas.

If you are asked to do this, it is worth putting some effort into it. There is no reason why you should not crib from whoever or whatever source you like – although if you do borrow heavily from others, it is wise to quote any published sources. Make sure what you write is readable and holds their attention. They may be judging your written communication skills as well as your ideas.

INTERVIEW ARRANGEMENTS FOR MANAGEMENT POSTS

For managerial posts, these are likely to be more elaborate – involving up to six panel members, and with each interview lasting an hour, sometimes more. A panel of six members is too large. The result is often poor co-ordination and little rapport with candidates. Moreover, people tend to ask their pet questions.

There are several reasons for having large panels. One is to give several important people the ownership of the decision. They may not say very much, but they have seen the candidate and agreed with the decision – or they may veto the decision of other panel members. For some posts, an external assessor may be present. The external assessor is the expert brought in from outside to assess the technical competence of the candidates, and also to give an objective external judgement, which is useful when people want to know how good internal candidates are. It is therefore fairly typical to find a more senior manager, a medical consultant, an external assessor and a personnel officer present with the recruiting manager.

Occasionally, there may be more than one round of interviews, with the first acting as a screening interview. The final interview will take place later on. However, time pressures are making this arrangement rarer, although you will sometimes be asked to attend two separate interviews, which are assessing different things.

For senior management posts, interviews can be very formal indeed. They are often held in austerely grand board rooms, usually reserved for disciplinary hearings and meetings of the authority. At this level, the probing can be deep – often of a person's management ideas. The probing of performance is often very inadequate, and a surprising high number of interviews at this level must be considered to be technically poor. A lot is read into the manager's ability to 'perform on the day', however good her track record may be. Coming across well in front of a bruising panel is often crucial for success. Panel members like to say 'We deliberately gave her a hard time. I like the way she stood up to us without being intimidated. That suggests that she will be a strong manager, not easily swayed.'

PSYCHOMETRIC TESTING

Another part of the series of events may be a psychometric testing session. The NHS has recently discovered occupational testing, which now enjoys a vogue for senior posts like unit general managers, district nurse advisers and senior college of nursing education posts. It does not seem to be spreading to lower levels yet. You will be asked to sit in a room and to undertake a series of pencil and paper exercises, usually taking up to half an hour each. Some will stretch your mind by asking you to solve problems. These are ability tests, which may reveal your capacity for verbal, numerical or abstract reasoning.

It is unlikely that selection will be based simply on how well people do in these tests. You may be expected to demonstrate a minimal level of reasoning ability, however.

If the job requires you to think quickly and draw conclusions accurately from verbal or numerical information, then it is appropriate to test this.

Pace yourself in these tests to give a good balance between speed and accuracy. Often, people who complete the test do not do as well as those who do fewer items, but do them correctly.

If personality inventories are used, they will indicate a pattern of personality traits, reveal how you relate to people, or show your preferred style of operating. In a well-researched test, the meaning of a particular score on a particular scale may be shown in relation to a given population – for example that you are more adaptable than 55% of managers. To use this information, the assessors will need to be sure that the score correlates with measures of success, or the known competencies of the job.

Quite often this research will not have been done, and in many cases the competencies will not be known for certain either. This means that the scores obtained cannot be definitive in the selection decision. The profile that emerges will be put together with other information to shed light on candidates' strengths and weaknesses. If candidates score an unacceptably extreme level on one of the traits measured, they may be rejected. It is unlikely that the assessors will have one ideal profile in mind. Occupational psychologists will often interview candidates to assist their interpretation of scores.

All candidates will face the temptation to present themselves in too favourable a light. There are three dangers in doing this.

Firstly, it could be picked up by the test and appear in the report as a tendency to lie, have poor self-perception, or as a desire to present yourself in a way that impresses others. Secondly, you may not be able to guess the meanings of items and the measures to which they relate. One test has an item asking if you like tall men. An affirmative answer here has nothing to do with social or sexual preferences. The third issue is whether it is wise to present yourself falsely. Let us say that the job calls for someone who is more assertive and better organised than yourself. If you secured the post, you might have problems. It might seem that you had been less than honest in describing yourself.

The use of personality inventories is not accepted by everyone. Some feel that they cannot do justice to the complexity and individuality of people. A list of scores on various traits may say little about someone's driving motivation and personal style, and may not do justice to the repertoire of behaviour that we all learn.

Results of tests are sometimes withheld from candidates, although they may be available on request. It will be up to potential employers to decide how much they disclose. Most would be prepared to disclose an individual's results to the individual, if asked, but would not give details of other people's on grounds of preserving confidentiality. This confidentiality could be breached, however, by order of an industrial tribunal looking for evidence in a case of unfair discrimination. If the information is kept on computer, it is covered by the Data Protection Act, and individuals will have a legal right of access to it.

ASSESSMENT CENTRES

Where a number of people are to be assessed for places – for instance, on a management development programme – it is not uncommon for candidates to be asked to perform a series of behavioural tasks and exercises as part of a selection process. The method is referred to as using an assessment centre (note that this is a method, not a place). A number of standard exercises, such as presentations, role plays, group discussions and negotiations, are designed. The candidates perform while being rated on a number of criteria. Those observing are trained to look for evidence of qualities such as leadership, ability to prioritise, sensitivity to others, communication skills and so on.

In assessment centres, actual performance is assessed directly. This is felt to be a more reliable guide to future performance than a less direct means of assessment, like an interview. Since each candidate is measured on a number of criteria by different observers in a number of tasks, a lot of information is available, and the effects of bias by the observer and of slight lapses by the candidate are minimised. Some qualities, such as resilience and creativity, are hard to assess by these methods.

Assessment centres tend to be used occasionally where the post is senior and skilled, where the competencies required are known, and where there is a large enough field of candidates to run group exercises. It can also be cost effective to run assessment centres where there are a large number of posts to be filled.

A prerequisite is the ability to simulate the requirements of the job in some sort of test exercise, and to train assessors to make consistent ratings. Needless to say, they are very expensive to develop and run, and if you are being invited to attend one, you can be sure that the ratings produced will be taken very seriously in the selection decisions. You may need to achieve an acceptable level of performance on each criterion on which you are being judged.

Hence, it will be useful to know, if you can, what the criteria will be. You will probably not be given prior details of the exercises, so you will not be able to rehearse your performance. But since presentations to an audience are very common, you would be wise to brush up your skills in this area. The main problem will be to keep going through all of the exercises. Find out, if you can, how many they are giving, whether there will be psychometric tests as well, and get a good night's sleep beforehand.

Information from the assessment centre will be quite detailed and will almost certainly be useful to you. However, unless you are an internal candidate, you may not be allowed access to it. Again, ask what happens to the data they have on you, and whether it might be used elsewhere, if you have any worries about this. Ask if you will be told the results.

THE TOUR

Quite often you will be offered a tour of the site on the interview day. Although intended to be useful to the candidate, such tours are often rushed and poorly planned, and do not give you much information, especially about the management of the organisation. You may get clues to staff morale and efficiency, how well organised things are, how up to date and how much cash is available.

Sometimes your host on the tour can be drawn to give you useful information. This person may be asked for an opinion on the candidates, and therefore it is recommended that you show enthusiasm and friendliness, and ask perceptive questions.

Negotiation of salaries or terms and conditions may take place. In the NHS, it is wise to raise, early on, questions about removal expenses or your desire to undertake studies and be funded by the district.

Do your homework beforehand on living arrangements. You may be judged as improvident or not a serious contender, if you have not.

Other matters, like starting dates, crown lease cars, holiday and training commitments, and the equipment you would like, can be left until you get the offer.

We know it will be a seller's market for people with professional or managerial skills in the next decade. The sophistication of selection methods, and their precision in predicting success, is likely to increase. These are hopeful signs for candidates.

Please do not imagine for one moment that you will secure any senior professional or managerial job without selling yourself. It will not be sufficient simply to write your qualifications and experience down on paper and assume that the selection process will be a formality. Whatever process is used, you will be actively assessed and expected to perform well enough to justify your claim.

Chapter 11

ASSORTED INTERVIEW HAZARDS

TWELVE IN A ROOM

Panels are sometimes far too big. For senior posts, it is felt a necessary ritual to ask everyone who could possibly have an interest to attend, perhaps to ask one question each (their pet question). Such interviews gather little in the way of evidence. I met someone who was 'interviewed' by all members of a local authority. Senior posts in new colleges of nurse education, for instance, may well require many political interests to be represented, and therefore necessitate large panels undertaking ritual questioning.

You may be asked, as I was, about a situation 10 years ago, and probed exhaustively about how you acted then. It is difficult to remember the detail in the first place, and also quite disconcerting for the panel to conclude that your actions would necessarily be identical *now*.

THE COMPANY OF WOLVES

Interviewers are often taught to explore gaps and discontinuities, and to probe deeply for any evidence of negatives in your life – like situations that did not work out or courses that you left before completion. Sometimes this can be difficult. They may constantly refer back to the negative side, and when you admit something like 'I found the pressure too much', the whole panel will sometimes attack your flagging form like a pack of wolves. 'Too much pressure, eh?', says one interviewer, 'Do you often find it difficult to cope with pressure?', continues the interviewer, perhaps with a smug feeling that she's really on to something here. Even if you truthfully say 'I can as a rule', you will not be believed, and this theme may well re-occur in other questions, 'Might you find some similar pressure in this job?'. A second interviewer might have picked up on this point as well, saying 'I'd like to pick up what you said to my colleague about coping with pressure. . .'. I have found it useful to take the line 'That was then and this is now. I have learned to cope since. How useful that experience was!'

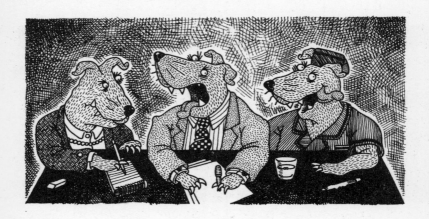

TWELVE IN A DAY

Be wary of the panel that has been working all day when you are finally called, an hour or so behind schedule, at 5 p.m. On one such occasion I remember missing out on the tour of the department that was to follow, because everyone else in the building had gone home.

Panels often give themselves too much work. This means they lose sharpness, they stop listening, they cannot remember who said what, and they cannot read their notes, which become more sketchy as the day goes on. Occasionally, you will find that an interviewer actually nods off during the interview.

You may find that you follow the candidate who seems just what they want. In such a situation, you may feel that they are just going through the motions with you. Interviewers always feel obliged to give you some chance to prove yourself, but it may be distinctly half-hearted.

FITTING IN AND FOBBING OFF

If you don't fit in, you are likely to be fobbed off. 'Fitting in' is the bane of selection. Everyone uses the term, most look for people who do, but few realise its potentially discriminatory power. Clearly, relating to the people that already work there is important, and nobody in their senses would pick a team of incompatibles. However, this may lead to people jumping to conclusions. If your potential colleagues differ in age, interests, gender and ethnic background, this is perhaps something you should be aware of, although you may enrich the team by being different. Let us say that the team is rather old and set in its ways, perhaps cliquish. You should be told (or see for yourself), and it may be reasonable to discuss this at the interview. But instead of this, people are often fobbed off on the lines of 'You wouldn't like it here', which is a veiled way of saying 'You wouldn't fit in'. So *all* the negatives are stressed, and it is hoped that you will say 'Well, no, I think you're right, that would be difficult for me. It's not really what I'm looking for.' The panel then breathes a sigh of relief. They have your admission, and their conscience is clear, even if you are the best qualified person ever to walk through their doors.

SOME OTHER DISCRIMINATORY PLOYS

I sat and observed an interview where a male interviewer was looking to see if the female candidate was wearing an engagement ring. She deliberately concealed it below the table. So he then started to ask whether she would have problems with the absences from home, which the job would require. What he really wanted to know was 'Are you getting married?' or even 'Are you thinking of starting a family' – questions that are rarely, if ever, asked of men. Female interviewers tend to be concerned with 'Who will look after the children if you are sick?'. There is still a belief that they will elicit the real truth on these issues from the interview, or that candidates to whom it applies will not have resolved this issue before coming for interview. If the issue is raised by the candidate, I would expect it to be pursued, but fairly.

If you are a female and get this kind of question, I suggest you stay cool, smile and then say 'I'm rather surprised that you felt it necessary to ask me that. Naturally, I wouldn't have considered applying if that was a problem for me. Perhaps you could explain its relevance to the post?'

THE HALO OR THE HORNS

These expressions refer to the tendency of panels to make strong positive or negative judgements of a candidate in one area, usually early on, and then to ignore all contradictory evidence. You are made out to be an angel or a devil, and from then on the interviewers seek evidence to confirm that. Often, the positive evidence is based on some similarity you have to the panel member. Maybe you went to the same school, or you hold the same views about nursing. If you acquire the horns, quite often by disagreeing with the interviewer's pet ideas, some will make a lot of effort to 'put you down' on other things, by asking you tough questions, or even by setting out to antagonise you. 'I know you may not agree with me, but don't you think you might be wrong?' is the tenor of the questioning. So you agree (and appear weak); or possibly disagree (and appear contrary). Having been put down in this way, you can be marked down. It is rather like the trial of witches.

Chapter 24 discusses some other kinds of bias.

Chapter 12

PERILS OF BEING AN INSIDER

With the changes taking place in management structures, many nurses may find themselves reapplying for their current posts under a new job title. Others may seek promotion where they are. In most cases, the process is much the same – completing the application form and, if shortlisted, attending the interview.

Two out of six candidates who applied for a newly created post in their own unit agreed to help throw some light on the process. They did not know until after the interview that they would be approached for assistance later.

Members of the interviewing panel were also happy to assist us. Chapter 23 presents their point of view.

The whole exercise was carried out with Sally Colter of the Raine Partnership. The Raine Partnership is a firm of consultants dealing with all aspects of recruiting in the health care industry, offering advice on careers, curriculum vitae and post-interview counselling, and specialising in senior management recruitment. For obvious reasons, the names and the place have been changed.

Case study 1

Michael Davis is in his forties, married with children of school age. He has worked at the Alberton Hospital since 1976, during which time he was promoted to charge nurse. He was not sure about applying for the two new posts created as a result of a change in care. His current grade is F, the new post is G.

Michael felt that the 24-hour commitment required by the new post holder would be more than he could manage because of his family. His wife works on night duty, and if he were called out at

---

night, the children would be unattended. However, he realised that if he didn't apply, he would automatically become deputy team leader. He would then have the same commitments when acting as team leader, but without the obvious advantage of the higher grade salary.

After much deliberation, and feeling very unconfident, he decided to accept management's invitation to apply for the job. Nevertheless, he resented the pressure put on him to go through this stressful procedure. Filling out an application form is a tedious job which most people find irksome, and Michael was no exception.

It is 13 years since he went through that process. 'I can't sell myself and I always underestimate what I am capable of doing', he said. He never considered the possibility of writing a formal curriculum vitae.

Because of his ambivalence over applying, Michael left completing the application form until very late. It was therefore hurried and handwritten. It contained the bare facts, but little thought went into presenting the information.

Michael made no preparations for the interview either. He felt it would be a form of 'cheating' to ask people who had recently been interviewed for other posts what to expect.

Most people feel nervous at the prospect of an interview, and Michael was no exception. 'I was tense the night before and nervous on the day. I felt as though I was going in front of a magistrate. I don't know why. I knew everyone there', he said.

Having an interview can feel like taking your clothes off in public. The interviewers examine you, warts and all. Many people find it even more uncomfortable being interviewed by people they know. This bothered Michael, who afterwards wondered what certain people must think of him.

The interview room – not the normal one – was informal, with low easy chairs surrounding a coffee table. However, Michael found himself facing a partly filled bookshelf behind the interviewers. This was distracting. The wall behind him was glass panelled and, although he could not see the passers-by, he was aware of them because of the changes in the light. He knew they could see what was going on and this made him feel uncomfortable.

Michael knew the interviewers, one man and three women. They put him at ease but Michael felt that the questions they asked him were very difficult. Because he had made no enquiries beforehand, he had no idea what they might ask, but assumed it would be related to the job description and about his work. He felt unable to explain himself properly and the interviewers did not help.

'They knew I was uncomfortable. They asked tough questions to make me feel worse, I think. They would ask one question and then something more difficult', he said. When he could not answer a question there was silence. This was particularly uncomfortable. 'You don't know whether or not you got the answer right or wrong', he said.

Two questions were particularly difficult. One was about equal opportunities. The other was about the difference between a manager and a leader. He had no idea what the questioner was looking for.

While Michael was being questioned by one panellist, others were writing. He found this very disconcerting.

At most interviews, candidates are given the opportunity to ask questions, but Michael was not prepared for this and had none to ask. In retrospect, he feels he should have done so. 'It makes the candidate look interested – it shows he is looking forward to the job', he commented.

Before he left the interview, Michael was asked whether he wanted to know the result by letter or telephone.

Michael felt the interview had gone badly immediately after it was over. He knew he had failed to get the job. 'I felt I had only given 60% of myself.' Nevertheless, he thought he had answered one question well. He was particularly disappointed about the way he had handled questions from his manager. 'She must wonder how I can do my job', he said. Had he been in her shoes he would have made allowances based on his knowledge of the candidate's work performance and perhaps seen him later when he was more relaxed.

However, he felt no animosity. 'The interviewers did a good job. I just did not prepare myself and thus the interview went badly.' Michael now realised he should have done his 'homework' before the interview – asking people what to expect.

Michael was not successful this time, but he had learned some lessons. He will never apply for a job again with a negative attitude. In future, he intends to be better prepared. He believes that nothing is a foregone conclusion. He has no regrets about applying, but could kick himself for not putting more effort into it. The experience, together with the valuable post-interview counselling he received from his manager, and from Sally Colter, has sharpened his ideas about himself, his skills and the job he does.

Post-interview counselling, the policy for this unit, was offered to Michael immediately he was told the result of the interview. Although he knew where he went wrong, it was helpful to have it pointed out by someone on the other side of the fence. 'Sally offered me positive encouragement and told me how to answer questions.'

Michael is determined to apply for any team leader post that comes up in the future. He is not interested in moving location because of his children's schooling and his wife's work commitments. He will seek advice on how to prepare a curriculum vitae next time. 'It never occurred to me that I should prepare myself or sell myself on paper at the interview', he said.

Despite the fact that he sees himself as a positive individual, he does not feel confident. He thinks he does his job well, initiates and organises ventures for the residents in his care and manages them well, but he has never analysed what skills are involved. This particular health authority offers one-day interview training, but Michael did not take up the opportunity. He now wishes he had.

Case study 2

Tony Brown is 40, also married with schoolchildren. He has worked at Alberton Hospital since 1972. In 1987, he was promoted to senior nurse, but because of management re-organisation he went back to ward work as a charge nurse on a protected salary.

Tony was very angry about the creation of the posts and the fact that there was only one instead of two designated leaders proposed for each team. He also felt that the whole selection process was a meaningless ritual. However, having decided to apply, he made an effort to present himself well in his written application. The section asking for a 'short account of relevant experience' was typewritten and clearly set out. Tony also did his homework well, asking colleagues who had been interviewed in the last year what he would be asked.

At the interview, he felt relaxed but inwardly angry. 'I didn't think I appeared angry at the time', he said. He felt good, but not confident that he would get the job. The competition was reasonably stiff, with six people being interviewed.

Tony found no problems with the interview room apart from the seating. He is a big man and the low easy chairs were uncomfortable, causing him to shift position frequently. The low seating also made him feel at a disadvantage.

'The interviewers were welcoming, and the first question posed by the educationalist would have put anyone at ease', said Tony. 'He asked me what I had been doing for the past two years. I think it was a beautiful start.' Most of the questions were, as he expected, related to the job description, and none were difficult. However, he was glad that he had done his homework. Like Michael, Tony found the question on the difference between a manager and a leader disconcerting. He answered that the two interlink, but there was a silence. 'I received no vibes as to whether or not my answer was satisfactory', he said. Finally, the silence was broken by a question from someone else, but he confessed 'It threw me for a while.' He has still no idea what the questioner was looking for.

Tony had not prepared any questions for the panel. Had it been an external interview, he would have done. However, he does not feel that it is important to ask questions as it gives the candidate some form of control over the proceedings.

On the whole, Tony thought he interviewed well. He felt he went over the top when he tried to inject some humour into one of his answers. But he believes humour, handled well, is important, and should be something the interviewers consider.

Tony felt that the interviewers did their job well. But he felt the interview was interminably long, probably because two candidates had dropped out earlier. 'It took 55 minutes. I kept looking at my watch because it was taking longer than I anticipated for a job at this level. I was glad when it was all over', he said.

Did he think he had got the job? 'No. And when I heard by telephone three to four hours later, there was no euphoria. I never felt so flat after a promotion in all my life', he said. Tony thought that the three women on the panel were less understanding of his behaviour than the man. He realised that, at one stage, he took control with one of the interviewers, firing questions at her, but it was not intentional.

Body language is very important, and Tony was told later by one of the interviewers that he had been stroking his beard, which gives 'bad vibes'. He felt that most people in that situation are not conscious of what they are doing.

Unlike Michael, Tony did attend the one-day workshop two years ago. He found it useful, although a bit rushed, with no time for proper feedback. Tony felt the selection feedback had been valuable. It had given him good interview experience and made him prepare a professional curriculum vitate for the future, which he would adapt to suit the appropriate job description.

Clearly, there were problems with these interviews which would not have occurred if the candidates had been external applicants. The political problems surrounding the creation of the posts had led to resentment and anger. And it is never easy to be put through a formal procedure by people you know well. Candidates often find it difficult to know how to behave and may present a false impression, surprising those conducting the interview.

Michael believes that, instead of using the normal selection procedure for internal applicants, managers should monitor their progress for a period of months and make a decision on their performances, with perhaps a less formal discussion at the end of that time. If formal selection procedures are seen to be necessary for internal posts, perhaps it would be helpful for both sides to have an external assessor on the interviewing panel.

The two candidates described here had the added advantage of a post-interview counselling session. Both men found the additional advice, from someone who was an impartial observer, invaluable.

Whatever the outcome of a job application, it is always a valuable experience. Having to analyse one's job and lifestyle, and face the potential consequences of changing the *status quo* does sharpen your thinking and shakes the nice comfortable rut many people dig for themselves.

For the unsuccessful candidate, the temptation is to go away and lick her wounds, but with good counselling, a negative experience can be turned into a positive one.

PREPARATION HINTS FOR INTERNAL CANDIDATES

Here are some of the things you need to think about as an internal candidate.

Find out what the interviewers are looking for

It does no harm to ask this question before the interview, if you are not sure. Get the job description and all the information you can muster about the new post. Ask other people what they think the job will entail. Remember that you may be too close to the situation to assess this objectively.

Find out what the selection procedure will entail

Quite often internal candidates are interviewed more or less as a courtesy, but there may be no commitment to appointing from within. If people are to be 'slotted in' to new posts as part of a re-organisation exercise, the position will be different from that of open competition. So you need to know what the rules are. Personnel officers and trade union stewards will be able to tell you what the rules are, and of your rights and obligations. If you are competing with external candidates, will the internal candidates be given first option? Will the selection process be the same for both?

Find out where you stand

You may or may not be able to secure an appraisal interview with your boss that might give you an understanding of your shortfalls. Somebody within the organisation should be honest with you about your chances. You will probably need to provide a reference. Internal candidates are sometimes encouraged to apply for posts because the boss wants them to get the experience of applying. The boss may not be sure whether you are ready for promotion, and so wants to have you assessed by others. This can lead you to some false expectations if you have not been told this.

Check if they have a stereotyped picture of you, as, for example, 'part of the furniture', 'too old', 'too young', 'wanting to move too quickly', etc. Really work on giving a more acceptable picture. Often, by creating a slightly different image with people before the interview, you can get people to take you more seriously.

Study the panel members' interests

Ask other people who have been interviewed about their experience.

Be aware of your own feelings – but do not let them get in the way

If you are anxious or feel angry about being asked to apply, this will invariably go against you. Sometimes candidates who have to apply for their own job come over as flippant and cynical, and fail to convince the panel that they are serious contenders. You will be asked questions by people you know. It may seem unreal, or a rather pointless ritual, but they will be serious, and therefore you must be. Answer the questions fully. You can acknowledge the fact that interviewers know you, but cannot say 'Well, I thought you would have known my views (or record) on that.' Sometimes the interviewers who know you will be prompting you to enable you to impress the ones who do not.

Do your preparation just as thoroughly as you would for an external job

See Chapter 9 for guidance on this. Show enthusiasm, and have some questions to ask.

Study the procedures that apply in internal re-organisations

You will have certain rights, obligations and choices. Be fully aware of them. There may be situations where the panel is going through the motions because the procedure requires it – or where the rules are conveniently forgotten.

Nothing should come as a surprise but do not assume that they will make things easy for you. The panel may fear criticism for appointing an insider, and therefore make it tough and make you prove your worth.

The following checklist summarises the steps involved when preparing for an internal interview.

Checklist 12.1

1 Find out what the interviewers will be looking for.
2 Study the selection procedure.
3 Find out where you stand.
4 Study panel members' interests.
5 Be aware of your own feelings.
6 Prepare as for an external interview.
7 Know the rules in internal re-organisations.

Chapter 13

ON THE DAY – THE INTERVIEW

There was things which he stretched, but mainly he told the truth.

Mark Twain, *Adventures of Huckleberry Finn*

DRESS AND APPEARANCE

It is important that you turn up looking smart and clean. They must think that you have taken some time and trouble for the interview. So if you have had to change a car tyre on the way because you have had a puncture, make sure that the hand you shake theirs with is clean.

GETTING THERE

You must be on time at all costs. Failure to do so will mean that

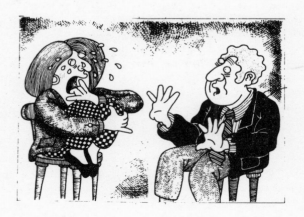

you will arrive flustered, and give a very bad impression. This will mean planning your journey. Aim to arrive 15 minutes early. If you are coming by public transport, check the times of buses and trains carefully, and allow for cancellations. If you are travelling by car, avoid the rush hour if you can, even if it means getting there early and having a cup of coffee before you go for the interview. Check that you have been sent a map, and that it is clear. There is nothing worse than traipsing around a large hospital, trying to get your bearings, in a state of panic because you are late. The following checklist lists the items that you should take with you.

Checklist 13.1

1 The job details.
2 A copy of your CV or application form.
3 The map and timetable.
4 Your own notes and questions to ask.
5 Something to read if you have to wait.
6 The telephone number and some spare change for a telephone call.
7 Some aspirins.

When you get there, find out where the loos are, and where the interview will take place. Check if they are running to time – usually they will be running late. If there is a briefing for all candidates to begin with, or if they are running late, you may be told that you will not be required until a certain time. This will give you the opportunity to rehearse your script, read your notes or a book, practise your relaxation techniques, or chat to the other candidates.

If you are allowed to chat to other candidates – some interviewers carefully keep them away from each other – you are advised not to get too deep into conversation. You might lose concentration, or energy, if you get into a deep conversation, and then you will have to readjust quickly to the interview situation. On the other hand, you may find it helpful to exchange a few pleasantries. It might reduce your anxiety and get you in the mood for talking to strangers. Internal candidates can often give you useful information, particularly about whether they have high expectations of getting the job. Do not expect them to give too much away, obviously.

MAKING YOUR ENTRANCE

We know that first impressions count for a very great deal. Once an impression is given, it lasts, and research suggests that interviewers will often be looking for evidence to support that initial judgement.

You will be dressed appropriately. However, it may be wise to avoid extremes – it is best to compromise. If two visits are required, do not wear the same outfit. If you always wear the same 'interview suit', it may come to be associated with failure.

You must walk in fairly confidently, but not arrogantly. Try to smile. You do not want to look like a grinning idiot, but you need to respond to their welcoming remarks fairly positively. You will immediately gauge how formal things are. Be ready to shake hands, as this is still the norm, and make direct eye contact, even though it is tempting to look around to discover where they want you to sit. If convenient to do so, close the door behind you.

It is important at this stage to try to listen to what is said. You will be introduced to the panel. Remember the names and the job titles. You may simply feel sickness in the stomach or a parched throat at this time. You must breathe deeply as you settle into the chair, and say to yourself under your breath 'relax'. By this time, you will be aware of who is in charge.

It is permissible to adjust the chair if it is too close. The best position is one where you can address all the people in the room without having to swivel or completely change your posture. Do say something if the sun is affecting you. No serious interviewer is trying to make you feel stressed by the environment.

BODY LANGUAGE

Here, you must try not to shake, or slump or fiddle with anything. Do not fold your arms. The best posture is an open one, where you appear to be listening, with as much eye contact as you can muster, but avoid giving a fixed stare. That can be quite threatening.

ANSWERING QUESTIONS

You can be sure that when questions are fired at you, in your nervous state, you will not be able to respond in anything like the way you may have intended. Hence, any practise of set answers is likely to be a waste of time. Even if you remember the words, you will sound stilted, possibly false. Make a conscious effort to speak up.

Some people dry up when they are nervous, others talk too much and tend to talk gibberish. When a question is asked, remember to give yourself time. This is the first lesson in keeping control. Say 'I need to think about that. . .' if you need to, or 'That's an interesting question' perhaps, to give yourself time to think. Then the pause can come naturally, and does not seem awkward.

Answer the question – unless you deliberately do not intend to. Do not be afraid just to say yes or no. The interviewer will prompt you to say more if she wants you to. Obviously, you will avoid making a string of monosyllabic responses, but equally annoying is the kind of person who must elaborate on every answer. If you are too long winded, you will see the interviewers showing signs of impatience. They may say 'Perhaps we can come back to that later. . .' or 'Yes, yes, yes, that's fine, can we move on now?'.

CONTROL

Control is about having breathing space and being able to take the interview in the direction you want it to go. You can create space for yourself by taking your time to answer, sometimes asking for clarification, or breaking up complicated questions in a way that makes it easier for you to answer.

So you may say, politely, 'I wonder if you could rephrase that question?', or 'I am not quite sure what kind of answer you want. . .'.

You can also say 'Let me answer that in this way. . .' to emphasise a particular slant that you might want to make. Or 'Can I take the second part first?'. Quite often they get so interested in your answer that the first part (which you weren't keen on answering) gets left behind and forgotten.

You will match your style to the interviewer's to some extent, but do not pander. If your interviewer is giving signals that she wants short, decisive answers, this is what you should give. But if you have reservations, it might be better to say 'Certainly, yes, in most circumstances. . .' (and then to explain any exceptions, if asked), rather than to say 'It all depends. . .' which will seem wishy washy. On the other hand, if your interrogator is inviting you to reflect, you might take more time to give a carefully considered response.

You can get control by obtaining permission. For instance, if you are given a question that you want to answer in a certain way, ask 'May I answer that by reference to. . .'. They will probably say 'yes' and you can then move into an area you feel confident in. Remember the interviewer controls the length of the interview, but the candidate, by the length of her answers, can control the number of questions asked in that time.

LEAVING THE RIGHT IMPRESSION

How to admit ignorance

Try at all costs to avoid sounding apologetic or, on the other hand, sounding arrogant. Real confidence is being able to admit ignorance at times, and not being ashamed of it. 'That's a very interesting question, isn't it!' brings out a knowing smile from the interviewer. Then, 'I'm not sure I know the answer to that' gains more respect than saying 'I don't know' in the first place, which does nothing for you.

Don't argue

Make sure that you do not get drawn into arguments. Some interviewers will try to draw you in, to see if you get rattled. If you decide not to commit yourself, or to pander to what you think the interviewer's views are, she might chase you off your fence and from one side to the other. So you must be firm, and sufficiently assertive, but not argumentative. You can always say something like 'That's my view, but I would admit that other views are worth considering' or 'Yes, you've got a point there' without losing face. Do not be too intense, or too flippant – but the right touch of humour will relax everyone.

If you do storm out of the room or end up in a blazing argument, you may live to regret it. You may want to reapply for another job in the same place, or come across your protagonist or one of her colleagues as an assessor elsewhere. Interviewers have long memories, and the bad impression you give in one place can damage your chances in another.

Don't deprecate

Do not criticise your current employer. They will automatically assume that you are disloyal. You can criticise the job, or say you feel you have outgrown it.

How am I doing? Do you agree with me?

Interviews are quite different from most normal conversations, in that you rarely get much idea whether or not you have said something pleasing to the interviewers. They are unlikely to say 'Yes, I totally agree' or 'We are impressed with your answers'. But it can happen, usually as some clever ploy by an interviewer who wants to lead you on so she can dramatically and disconcertingly stop you short with 'But that's not the whole story, is it?'. One must live with this lack of response, and do without the kind of reinforcement and endorsement that you might want. You will, of course, get head nods, but these will not necessarily signify endorsement of what you are saying.

You will find that some panel members may say nothing at all. Usually, they are not meant to, and have agreed to leave the questioning to others. They will probably be silently judging you. This spectral presence disconcerts some candidates. It should not, if you can establish some non-verbal rapport, as you might with a foreigner in a railway carriage.

WHEN YOU GET THE OFFER

Normally, you will leave on good terms, having asked when and how you might hear the result. Some candidates are asked at the end of the interview whether they would accept the post if offered it. You really have to say 'yes' at that point, even if you have some reservations or conditions still to negotiate.

If you are lucky, you will get that telephone call, offering you the job. You might be able to say 'yes' right away, having done all your homework thoroughly. If you are still not sure that it is the right move, however, you will need to ask for some time to make up your mind. If you have serious reservations, it is a good idea to ask to talk to the person who will have telephoned you quite soon afterwards. Say 'There are still one or two things I need to clarify. Perhaps we could meet very soon to discuss them?'

I have heard of posts where the interviewee is called at one day's notice and expected to give a 'yes' or 'no' answer instantly. It is never unreasonable to ask to sleep on it. You might say 'I think I will say yes, but I would just like a little more time. Perhaps I can ring you tomorrow' (or whenever).

If you have agreed to attend a job interview elsewhere within a few days, you may want to negotiate an extension of the time to allow you to make up your mind.

Maybe you have completely oversold yourself at the interview. You may realise that you will never live up to the lies you have told, and seek the quickest possible escape. You may want the job, but feel the need to soften the expectations of the person who has offered it to you. Again, an early meeting will be appropriate.

You may be simply waiting to negotiate your terms. Be clear in advance what sort of deal will be acceptable to you. You might want removal expenses, for example, a lease car or hospital accommodation, or the chance for paid study leave. You are normally in a strong negotiating position if they have set their heart on you for a senior post. If you are more junior, they may be less keen to do business on these lines. Although there are policy regulations in most health authorities, rules can often be bent, especially for people taking up senior positions. You should get any offer in writing, as you may need the proof that you have been offered the chance to do a higher qualification if there is a freeze on study leave after you join.

You may also need to negotiate your starting date, after discussion with your existing employer.

If you decide to accept the offer, you should write a letter of acceptance confirming that you are looking forward to joining them on such and such a date. If you have had a request accepted at the interview, or been offered anything over and above the stated terms and conditions, it is important to refer to this again in your letter in terms such as 'I am accepting the post subject to the offer of. . . Please let me know immediately if my understanding of this is not correct.'

If some contractual points are still unclear, or there are other conditions you want to secure, it is best to arrange a further meeting and ask for the outcome to be put in writing. Many people feel resentful when a promise or impression given at the interview is later denied.

IF YOU DON'T GET THE OFFER

Do you really want to know why? Do you need to know why? It may be that you do not care to know, or that it was so obvious that you would be embarrassed to ask. However, you may want to know why you were not the preferred candidate, or maybe not good enough in their opinion to do the job, or simply did not convince them by your presentation. All of these might be relevant.

If you simply ask why you did not get the job, you may get a panegyric about the qualities of the successful candidate, which you could not have matched in a month of Sundays, or someone telling you all of the weaknesses the panel detected, or a panning of your interview style. I recommend that you say something like 'Would you be good enough to tell me the reason why X was chosen over me. It would help me to know if I was applying for the wrong job or simply need to improve my presentation.' It will help if you can reassure the person you speak to that you are not criticising the decision.

If you then get a genuine response, you can decide on the level of detail you need to have. Bear in mind that it is not easy for most interviewers, who do not know you, to discuss your failure with you. Make it easy for them to help you, by being open and not resentful or angry in any way. Do not react to the well-meant criticism you will get. Remember it is bound to be useful to you, even if only as an example of how some interviewers think and make judgements. In Chapter 25, we look in detail at the interviewer's task in this.

SUSPICIONS OF DISCRIMINATION

If you suspect unfair discrimination, you may want to make notes on all the details that suggest this. Was there any obvious discrimination? Were you fobbed off? Was the post offered to someone with less relevant experience or inferior qualifications?

You can only take a legal case against the employer if it is on the grounds covered by the Race Relations Act or Sex Discrimination Act, or on the grounds of your trades union activity. See Chapter 19 for a discussion of unlawful discrimination.

Most personnel officers will take a case of possible discrimination seriously, and they will normally feel obliged to carry out some form of investigation. Since they work for the employer, you might question their objectivity, but they certainly would be keen to avoid legal action.

The Commission for Racial Equality or the Equal Opportunities Commission, or your union officer, will advise you. Bear in mind that it will be extremely difficult to get proof of discrimination, going to court can be a very lengthy and stressful business, and it is unlikely to get you the job you wanted.

Unless you feel you have a valid reason for taking up a serious grievance on the decision, I would advise you to lose gracefully – there may be a next time, and diplomacy will be advisable. Even if you think that the whole procedure was a complete shambles, you are probably best to keep that opinion to yourself, and perhaps one or two friends.

The following checklist will help you to prepare for the interview.

Checklist 13.2

1 Dress and appearance:
   - Be dressed appropriately – compromise.
   - Look smart and clean.
2 Getting there:
   - Be on time.
   - Make final preparations calmly.
   - Use relaxation techniques.
3 Making your entrance:
   - Enter confidently.
   - Try to smile.
   - Listen to what is said.
   - Remember names and titles.
   - Note who is in charge.
   - Make yourself comfortable.
4 Body language:
   - Keep still.
   - Make eye contact without staring.
5 Answering questions:
   - Speak up.
   - Give yourself time to answer.
   - Do not be thrown by the unexpected.
   - Answer the question asked.
   - Pick up feedback when you can.

---

6 Leaving the right impression:
   - Admit ignorance wisely.
   - Don't argue.
   - Don't deprecate.
   - Be enthusiastic.

REFERENCE

Equal Opportunities Commission, *Equal Opportunities: A Guide for Employees* (EOC, 1975).

FURTHER READING

Tschudin, Verena, *Managing Yourself*, Essentials of Nursing Management series (Macmillan, 1990).

Part Two

THE SELECTOR

In this part, we look at the interview from the other side of the table. We can do this by continuing the story we started in Part One, where Sally was being interviewed for a senior staff nurse post, grade E. As the story unfolds, the reader might like to think about the effectiveness of the interview process I describe. Although I have deliberately exaggerated to make my point, it contains many elements that are common in selection interviews. The faults are not, of course, confined to nursing selection.

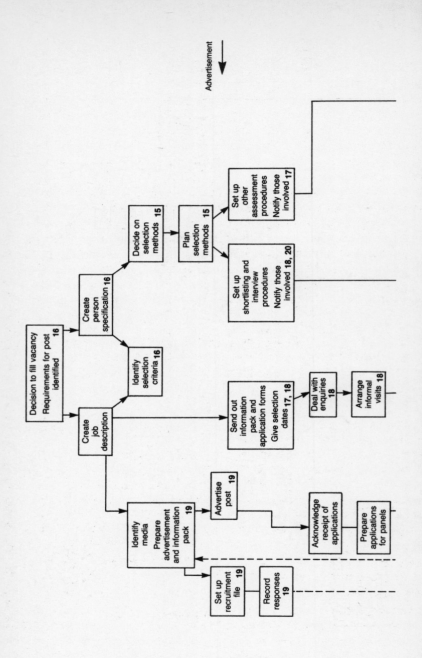

Advertisement

Decision to fill vacancy
Requirements for post identified **16**

Create job description

Create person specification **16**

Decide on selection methods **15**

Plan selection methods **15**

Set up other assessment procedures
Notify those involved **17**

Set up shortlisting and interview procedures
Notify those involved **18, 20**

Identify selection criteria **16**

Send out information pack and application forms
Give selection dates **17, 18**

Deal with enquiries **18**

Arrange informal visits **18**

Identify media
Prepare advertisement and information pack **19**

Advertise post **19**

Acknowledge receipt of applications

Prepare applications for panels

Set up recruitment file **19**

Record responses **19**

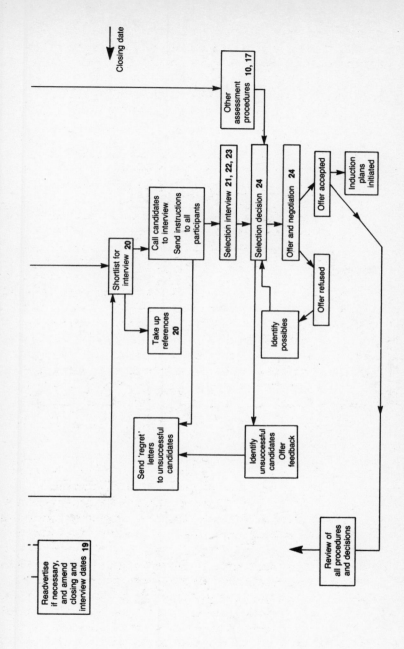

Flowchart B *The selection process for the selector* (numbers refer to chapters)

113

THE DAY OF JUDGEMENT – THE RITUAL

You will remember that we left our candidate in the hands of her interrogators.

The interview started with a few predictable pleasantries. Mrs Garnett then went on to ask Sally about her career to date. These were factual questions and quite easy for Sally to answer. However, Sally was not sure how much detail to go into. Mrs Garnett did not seem to know what to do to stop Sally. She kept smiling and nodding, in a shy friendly way. As she talked, Sally noticed that the tips of her fingernails were stained from the cigarette she had just been smoking. It was probably on her breath too.

Every so often there was an awkward pause. Mrs Garnett seemed almost as nervous as Sally was. The conversation did not seem to be going anywhere. Sally found herself talking about the difficulties she had had in one job, and out of the corner of her eye she noticed Miss Williams pull out a pen and make notes. This disconcerted Sally, who dried up as soon as she did so. Mrs Garnett seemed to be running out of questions. She was asking questions with obvious answers, like 'Would you mind taking charge?', 'Are you confident about your clinical knowledge?', 'Could you cope with the pressure here?'. She seemed to be revealing some of the questions in her mind, speaking out loud, rather than probing Sally's competence.

Miss Williams began to break the silences with her own questions, which were always sceptical ones, like 'Have you really had any experience with that kind of patient?', 'Don't you think you have forgotten some important aspects?'. Besides having to conduct two different conversations at once, each with a different tone and purpose, Sally had to swivel her head round to maintain eye contact.

Miss Williams was more confident in her questions, but by no means friendly. She felt that Miss Williams was looking for her faults, rather than her good points.

Sally had mentioned that she had had a poor relationship with a sister in a surgical ward during training, and had consequently failed an assessment. Sally was sorry she had mentioned this, as Miss Williams seemed to be making the assumption that Sally had been unwilling to listen to the sister's advice, and this was the reason for her failure. In fact, the sister had been a poor teacher, and Sally had been unwell at the time. But when she offered these reasons, they only made things worse. Miss Williams seemed to be inferring that Sally tended to blame others for her own failings. Her sickness record was also raised in a fairly confrontational way.

Miss Williams looked at Sally with a cold, fixed gaze. After her replies, Sally felt a sharp silence, as if the space was being left for her to fill it with some unguarded remark, and thus reveal further apparent flaws. Instead of saying something impressive, Sally ended up mumbling and starting sentences she could not finish.

'How do you see yourself in five years' time?', said Miss Williams.

'I can't be sure about that at the moment', said Sally. Again, this was the wrong thing to say, but if she had said that she wanted to be at Miss Williams's level, that would have sounded cocky.

Miss Williams posed a number of imaginary clinical situations and asked Sally how she would deal with them. Sally was afraid of saying the wrong thing. 'I'm not sure...' she said, knowing this would appear indecisive. Miss Williams rephrased the question another way. Sally was still perplexed. Further imaginary situations were presented to Sally. Once or twice she had come across the situation, or had seen the answer in a textbook. Several times the question seemed to be a catch question, and Sally ducked answering it.

Then, after about 15 minutes, the interview seemed to be all but over. It had lost its purpose. They were asking a lot of stock questions and seemed to have lost any real interest in Sally. They talked more and more, and she less. They were emphasising Sally's lack of experience and the difficulties she would have in the job. At that point, she knew she had blown it. She started to tell herself that she did not really want to work there anyway.

Sally was right about the reaction to her. After she had left, Miss Williams indicated that she had found this young lady wanting. Despite the attempt to gloss over her faults, Miss Williams felt she had detected them. Everything pointed to the fact that Sally was not of the calibre required, certainly not up to the standard of the person they had seen last week. A pity, but there it was – all the evidence pointed one way.

*   *   *

The interviewers had decided in two minutes, before the interview, the areas of questioning. 'You cover the application form and I'll cover clinical knowledge...'. They then called in the candidate and launched into the interview, hoping that something significant might show up.

116

They did not discuss the qualities they wanted, the criteria or the standards. They did not discuss how they were going to get evidence. They probably had some intuitive or stereotyped ideas of the person they were looking for, but they did not make them objective, and we did not know whether they shared these ideas. Any criteria they did use were in their heads, and they might have found it difficult to articulate them. They never discussed the candidates in relation to criteria, but merely compared one person with another, in rather vague subjective terms. Impressions were allowed to rule their judgement.

At the end, their decision was based on a very subjective reaction. It included some untested assumptions about the candidate. They thought they had evidence, but they ended up merely trying to justify their initial subjective impressions.

Candidates find their interviews rather random and unstructured. Apart from the use of certain pet questions, there is no common pattern between one interview and another. Their style is certainly idiosyncratic.

Shirley Garnett prefers to keep to factual information, but is not sure how to evaluate the information she receives. She certainly does not probe the candidate. She really would admit that she has little basis for selection. 'Why do I choose this one rather than that one? I am not really sure. As she has given better answers to my questions, I think she would be rather more organised on the ward.' Candidates often do not know what to make of her questions. Sometimes they are very leading, and the candidate is being invited to say the right thing. Sometimes candidates dry up because they do not know what she is getting at. Her inferences are hesitant and never tested.

Miss Williams, on the other hand, is highly judgemental. She regularly finds herself going beyond the factual evidence. She makes inferences and relies a lot on 'gut reaction'. This, for her, is her special art – weighing people up. It is what makes her a good interviewer in her opinion. 'There was something about that last candidate that I did not care for – perhaps it was her style of dress. She seemed a bit too forward – I am sure she would have given us trouble.'

Some candidates sense her hostility and are inhibited, or less than enthusiastic, in their replies. Miss Williams believes in putting a lot of pressure on people she feels are suspect, so that their faults are revealed – they get irritable or timid when she pierces their defences. She stares at them with cold eyes and pins them with questions. 'I knew she would crack if I pressed her hard enough – and I was right. She was not my kind of person. I think she was a bit sullen.' These self-fulfilling prophecies of a person with deep prejudices masquerade as real evidence.

Neither of the interviewers were aware of their mistakes, and they probably would not have much idea what to do about them, if they did know. Miss Williams would claim considerable skill and experience, but this claim has never been assessed. There is no system to her approach and no checks. Miss Williams's prejudices are unbridled. On the other hand, candidates know exactly what to say to impress Mrs Garnett. There is a lot of confrontation but no factual probing in her style.

A lack of precise and objective judgement may not matter too much. Perhaps the staff nurses they employ will have a good basic training and any faults they have will not be critical. Some good people might be rejected, but this will not matter if there is a good supply of capable people. This might not be the case in the near future.

Chapter 14

PERSPECTIVES FOR THE SELECTOR

THE SURVIVAL OF INTERVIEWING

In all the years that people have been selected for jobs, it is unfortunate in some ways that some method other than the interview has not become popular. Psychologists are always telling us not to rely on the interview for selection – they can prove that interview judgements are often poor. Everyone can do it badly – but this is never brought home to people, except in the case of their disasters.

Everyone wants to do interviews. There is an understandable compulsion to meet the people who will be working with us, and this leads us easily to want to turn this meeting into an

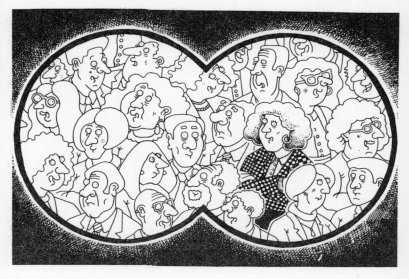

assessment procedure. So the meeting becomes a 'conversation with a purpose', and the tradition shows no sign of disappearing.

However, unlike other conversations with a purpose, like a clinical interview, the job interview has become a rather frightening ritual, where neither side is particularly natural, and the candidate often does not do justice to herself. We all know really competent people who come over like idiots at job interviews. We all know very clever people whose interviewing style is hopeless. If the interview is going to persist as a selection device, and it will until something better comes along, everyone must seek to develop the same level of competence that they would expect to have in a clinical or professional role.

Traditions have made the average nurse reluctant to market herself to employers and to sell herself at the interview. In the commercial world, the emphasis has been on assertive, competitive self-promotion – even to the extent of overselling oneself – and of hard negotiation about terms being offered. In the world of nursing, on the other hand, the interview has been more like an extension of clinical assessment, and the terms and conditions have definitely not been negotiable. Many nurses have been conditioned to feel inadequate in interviews. For some, the fear of assessment makes them neurotic.

Many nurse managers have had no proper training, and are nervous, often as much as candidates are. They tend to conduct the interview as if it were a clinical assessment, or approach it intuitively. Given a knowledge of sound procedure, and a systematic approach, it will be relatively easy for them to use their existing skills to carry out a job interview confidently and well.

THE JOB SEARCH IN THE NINETIES

Whatever has happened in the past, all the trump cards will be held by the candidate from now on. There will be an insatiable demand for qualified people, and particularly for nurses.

Conroy and Stidston's research has indicated that there will be a reduction of 31% in the numbers of school leavers between 1983 and 1993. It is reasonable to assume that the NHS will suffer a proportionately greater reduction than this.

There has been a reduction of almost 30% in the numbers entering nursing training over the period. This allows for the reduction in pupil nurses, but also incorporates a 10% reduction in student nurses. Numbers had even begun to decline in 1982/3, which was the peak year for school leavers.

Another key characteristic of the NHS is its reliance on a very highly qualified workforce – which constitutes only 18% of the labour market. Estimates of the workforce in the Oxford Region alone suggest that one-half would have obtained five 'O' levels and above. The extent to which the NHS can continue with current expectations of attainment is questionable.

Given these factors, and the increasing demand for qualified staff, it has been estimated that one out of every three appropriately qualified females would have to be recruited for the NHS in 1993 – an impossible task. Competition within the 'service sector' will also be increasing.

Recruiting more males, part-time staff and mature entrants might help, but will not provide solutions. Urgent attention will need to be given to retention of staff and to the mix of skills required.

The implications

For the candidate

At first sight, this is good news for candidates – a wider choice of opportunities and very much a 'seller's market' for qualified people. However, this might raise some problems for them. There is bound to be some high-powered and persuasive marketing of jobs. Even mediocre ones will be dressed up in all kinds of fancy wrapping. Not only is there likely to be a vast range of vacancies, there may also be a bewildering variety of inducements to fill them. Mature employees and part-timers, including working mothers, will find employers taking their needs much more seriously – the horizons open to them will expand rapidly. Hence the need for candidates to be clear what they want.

Given the shortage of skilled labour, the candidates you want to attract will be able to sell their skills to employers outside the health sector. If you look at the summary on page 20 of the skills used by nurses, you will find that they are many and varied, and extremely useful to employers.

For the employer

Undoubtedly, there will be greater competition for scarce,

professionally qualified staff. People will start to spend more money, to make jobs more attractive and market them better. As an employer, you will feel the need to offer inducements to attract new staff, and to hang on to existing staff. You will also need to offer education and other opportunities.

There will be a need to attract more male staff and more mature staff. You will need to go out of your way to make jobs flexible and attractive to part-timers, who will be much in demand everywhere.

Some employers may lower their selection standards – and certainly some will redesign jobs to enable less skilled people to do the work that has to be done. This means, incidentally, that the professional staff will be expected to supervise these less skilled people and to teach them – putting a greater premium on these particular skills.

For the recruitment and selection process

The balance of power will change. This will probably not affect the way many employers do things. Many will still keep candidates waiting, and give them little chance to ask questions. They will not allow candidates to negotiate the conditions of work that are important to them, like flexible hours or access to certain facilities and training.

However, candidates will increasingly be able to pick and choose their employers, and the ones that adapt to this fact, by offering candidates access and choices, will be the winners. One indication of this is likely to be the increasing perception of the selection process as a two-way affair and as an open process.

If professional staff are hard to come by, one strategy might be to dispense with selection altogether. However, if it is going to require such effort and expense to find qualified staff, and to lure them away from other hungry employers, it might seem rather important to pick the right ones – people whose motivation will be right for that particular job, or whose performance will be adequate.

So it would seem that, even if employers are less fussy (that is, have lower selection standards), there will be a need to ensure 'value for money', and that the selection process itself does not turn people away or give them a bad reputation. As an interviewer, your skills will need to be good.

THE KEY PROCESSES

If you have read Part One, you will be familiar with the key processes. In fact, the processes involved in selection are similar for both candidate and selector.

Investigation

Both parties will need to do some preliminary investigation in some depth, to be sure they know what they each want. For the candidate, it will be to investigate her own requirements, the job market and the situations she is applying for.

The selector needs to be sure of her requirements; to identify where candidates with the right qualities can be found; and to assess their claims to have what is required. Perhaps less obvious is the need to investigate what might attract and retain them – that is, to investigate the candidate's needs. In a seller's market, this should not be overlooked.

If you are familiar with the notion of clinical investigation, you will realise that a systematic, thorough and critical approach is needed. This book will provide you with plenty of guidance to the right diagnosis.

Marketing

As the employer, you will need to market the organisation and the post on offer, and also yourself as a colleague or boss. This must be done both on paper and in person.

Both employer and candidate need to consider their presentation to each other, to ensure that their meeting will be worthwhile.

Matching

Although the interview itself is always seen as a process of selection for the employer, who has set it up to assess candidates, the candidate does also of course make an assessment of employers. This choice is going to be of increasing importance from now on. The matching process may also involve negotiation, to ensure that each party's needs are going to be met.

Matching implies that criteria have been set, against which a person or a job can be matched. Again, this should not be unfamiliar territory for people in clinical practice involved in assessment.

Evaluation

Evaluation is the outcome of a systematic matching process, based on objective criteria. It should be basically a rational decision, although most would allow some scope for intuition at times. Instead of evaluating a person's suitability for discharge or rehabilitation, for example, you will be evaluating whether your needs will be met by the person concerned.

Evaluation is a two-way process, in that both parties will make judgements about whether the other party is offering what they want. If the quest is unsuccessful, then either side may want to ask why, in order to do better next time.

You need to be more sure of what you are importing, because mistakes can have expensive consequences, and the more senior the post the worse the problem. You need to know that you can detect the qualities and skills you require, which presupposes that you know what you are looking for.

REFERENCE

Conroy, Margaret and Stidston, Mary, 2001 – The Black Hole – An Examination of Labour Market Trends in Relation to the NHS (NHS Regional Manpower Planners' Group, 1988).

FURTHER READING

Herriott, P, Recruitment in the 90s (IPM, 1989).

Chapter 15

SELECTION BASICS

SPECIFY THE REQUIREMENTS

This is the key to everything that follows. You must specify your requirements as clearly and concretely as you can to begin with. You need to have some fixed yardsticks – or criteria – to judge candidates by. Do they come up to your standard on the experience you think the job needs? Would the person be able to handle the pressures of the job?

Many people go into an interview thinking that a candidate can somehow be measured by using a job description. Yet, the job description is really just a list of tasks and says very little about the characteristics that may be required. Look at any job description for a job you do not know. Can you say, for example, where tenacity and tact may be required? Or whether really good communication skills are needed? Or motivation to work without much praise or reward from the medical staff?

CRITERIA NEED TO BE RELEVANT AND ASSESSABLE

It is important to check that the appropriate criteria have been identified – by studying the requirements of the job, a process known as job analysis – and that the criteria you have identified as important turn out to be the things that matter in practice. The latter – validation – is usually neglected, with the result that impressions are allowed precedence over the facts.

The following example lists some fairly typical selection

criteria. But do they provide a good enough standard? Are they criteria that you would want to use? Are they assessable from an application form or through interview?

Example

1 Must be well-motivated:
   What does this cliché mean? It can be interpreted in a number of different ways. Some will infer a particular motivation; some might think that any strong motivation is sufficient. Any candidate worth her salt will rehearse her answer to 'Why do you want the job?', so you have to be more subtle and more specific here.

2 Must have 3 'A' levels:
   This might be an essential requirement to start training, but where it isn't, are you not excluding people who might be bright but lack the magic qualification? Are you specifying an educational standard? If so, is this the most appropriate one? From now on, we shall be recruiting more nurses from Europe who are unlikely to have 'A' levels.

3 Must be good with figures:
   To what standard must the person be 'good' with figures? A pencil and paper test would seem more appropriate than an interview for assessing this criterion. Most candidates would be horrified to be asked mental arithmetic questions in the middle of an interview!

4 Must be able to get on with Mr Jones:
   If Mr Jones is a difficult consultant, then it probably is an important requirement. But how can it be tested, unless you put candidates with Mr Jones for a week? It would be better to specify what it is that is required – perhaps a high level of interpersonal skills, or supreme efficiency, or brilliant clinical nursing skills, or a certain way of thinking?

5 Must have leadership potential:
   Another cliché? Can you determine this in an interview? You might be able to detect it by exploring the candidate's achievements – Are they solitary or has she led others? Asking 'What is leadership?' is not going to give you the information you want.

6 Must have relevant experience:
   This is surely self-evident. You must specify what range and depth of experience is acceptable, and thus what is not.

The next chapter goes into the process of identifying requirements and setting criteria.

USE GOOD METHODS FOR GATHERING EVIDENCE

You need to get information about the person that relates to the criteria you set. This means that you have to have some way for collecting the evidence and for assessing it. Everything you know about a person is usable. What is in the application form and the references is evidence. The interview is a device for collecting evidence, but not the only one. In Chapter 17, we look at the options here, and how the interview fits into an overall selection strategy.

DEVELOP OPERATIONAL SKILLS

Selectors, especially interviewers, need to have the skills and confidence to operate the process and obtain the evidence they need from it. This means basic training in good practice and feedback on how they are carrying out the process. It may be that the method used is not capable of generating very good results in the first place – and I am afraid the interview has an impressive list of detractors – but nothing will work at all in the wrong hands. Because the interview seems such a natural human process, it is susceptible to all of the biases of which human beings are capable.

There is a lot of information in this book about how to interview, see particularly Chapters 20 and 21, and this is based on what is considered the best practice. It is also useful to study what psychologists have said about the limitations of the interview, and an awareness of the research can help to avoid obvious pitfalls.

MAKE SOUND JUDGEMENTS AND EVALUATIONS

Assuming that you know what you are looking for, is all of the information you collect equally useful as a measure of the person's suitability? You need to know what to take seriously, and what to ignore. You need to extricate your own biases and prejudices from the facts. The interview gives both sides scope for generating information that is unreliable as evidence. In Chapter 24, we look critically at these issues. Chapter 24 discusses issues related to errors of judgement.

THE SELECTION CONTEXT

No selection method will work unless attention is paid to the detail. You need to be aware of selection as a total process, and not simply think about the interview. Chapter 18 provides a guide to the whole process, which is summarised in flowchart B on page 113.

Attention to detail is required in all of the processes – investigation, marketing, matching and evaluation – which were discussed in Chapter 14.

CONSIDER THE IMPACT ON CANDIDATES

Besides the public relations aspects of your selection process, you also need to be aware of the choices that candidates have to make, and a good selection process will allow scope for this. The question of offering counselling and feedback is also something to which you must give attention. This is covered in detail in Chapter 25.

Figure 15.1 summarises the selection basics.

FURTHER READING

Heriott, P, Ed, *Assessment and Selection in Organisations* (Wiley, 1989).
Jackson, Matthew, *Recruitment Interviewing and Selecting: A Manual for Line Managers* (McGraw-Hill, 1972).

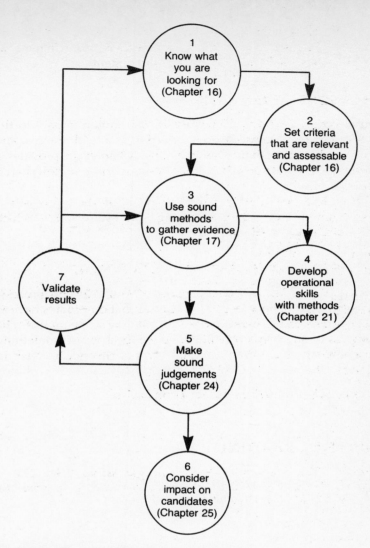

Figure 15.1   *Selection basics summary chart*

Chapter 16

CLARIFYING THE REQUIREMENTS

WHAT IS NEEDED?

The first reaction

When a valued member of staff leaves, there is a sense of loss and anxiety. The manager has to come to terms with the short-term problems and think about how to find the right replacement.

The panic reaction is to rush out and advertise for someone with similar attributes who will do an identical job. A more sensible response is to stand back and consider the future job requirements.

The need for change

The previous job description will usually give an inaccurate picture of the work that was being done. Perhaps the last person was with you for a long time and made the job her own. She may have taken on tasks beyond her normal duties, or avoided doing the things that she was not good at. Now there may be new demands or a need for a new emphasis in the work.

You may want to give the job more interest or change the level of technical skill. Perhaps you want to change the job content of other staff members, or move towards a new structure or regradings. You may need to merge responsibilities or even leave the post vacant for a while, until your aims can become clearer.

Involving the work team

If you involve the work team in the process of review and job design, you will almost certainly find that the members have ideas about what is needed. They may not have had the opportunity or courage to express them before. They will also be helpful as a sounding board for your own ideas. Bringing them into the discussion will alleviate their anxieties and give them a stake in the plans for the future.

You will find that they bring realism into your visions. They may comment on the job description ('This is far too much for one job') or the person specification ('You won't find this person on this earth'). From their knowledge of the job market, they can give advice on how to attract the right candidate. They might suggest that you introduce flexibility, novel recruitment methods ('This would be a good post for job share') and so on.

Producing a job description

New posts generate a great deal of excitement and interest. People make assumptions that duties in the new post will solve their own particular problems. It is important that the responsibilities are clarified, written down and agreed, or misconceptions are bound to occur.

Identify the tasks that have to be done, and the results required, with a picture of the situation in which the person will be working clearly in mind.

The process must be carried out early on, and certainly before the post is advertised. The published job description and details of your requirements give signals to the candidate. If they are woolly and vague, the candidate will assume that the organisation is like that too. If you are explicit about what you want, unsuitable candidates will be less likely to apply.

The full job description is likely to have the following sections:

- job title, salary and grade
- location
- reporting relationships
- job purpose
- key result areas
- tasks and duties
- qualifications, experience, skills and abilities required.

131

You will need to be clear about competencies (see later) when you set your selection criteria. Many people derive the selection criteria from the job description, but the problem here is that it is hard to identify competencies from a list of tasks (see page 125). Hence, you need to arrange your job description in such a way as to make the competencies stand out in relation to the tasks. You can then be much more precise in the section 'Qualifications, experience, skills and abilities required'.

You can do this by giving the 'Tasks and duties' section a clear structure, based on an analysis of the broad job roles. The following example shows you how this can be done for a clinical post.

Example

A nursing post will normally comprise roles such as practitioner, researcher, teacher or manager... of nursing care. Each role is likely to consist of component activities requiring one or more statutory nursing competencies, as defined in Rule 18 of the Nurses, Midwives and Health Visitors Rules Approval Order 1983 – Statutory Instrument 1983 No. 873 (see Appendix 2). Here is an example:

Role: Practitioner

Component	*Competencies*
1 Assess nursing needs.	Rule 18(i), (c) and (d)
2 Plan nursing care.	Rule 18(i), (e)
3 Implement nursing care.	Rule 18(i), (f)
4 Evaluate nursing care.	Rule 18(i), (g)

Use these component activities as subheadings and group the job tasks under each; for example:

Practitioner, Component activity 4: Evaluate nursing care
- (i) Assess the quality of care given.
- (ii) Assess patient achievements.
- (iii) Discuss achievement of care goals with colleagues.
- (iv) Identify improvements necessary.
- (v) Make changes as appropriate to nursing care plans.

Describe the tasks involved in all of the component activities within each role you have identified. These descriptions of tasks can include references to specific patient groups, techniques, procedures, programmes or locations, if you want them to – or they can be left general.

The *teaching* role will involve competencies described in Rule 18(f) and the teaching of the other competencies. The *managerial* role will centre on Rule 18(i) and include the integration of others' activities, as well as general or non-clinical managerial tasks. Where the duties involve a greater level (or range) of continuing responsibility, or the practice of more specialist competencies, this will often have a bearing on the clinical grading of the post. Such features should be clearly visible in your description of the tasks and duties.

Be careful, however, that tasks that do not fit neatly into the clinical categories are also included, like 'To order equipment and supplies, to ensure health and safety requirements are met, to complete Korner returns, to manage ward budgets...'. Some of them will fit under the 'manager of nursing care' role, while others will not and will require a miscellaneous 'Other duties' section.

If you are starting from scratch, and have established the context of the job, you will need to decide how much detail you need to state. It is better to concentrate on key activities than to produce a long undifferentiated list of tasks.

Use a consistent verb form of sentence, like: to ensure that...; to co-ordinate...; to supervise...; to report.... Words like 'to liaise...' or 'to be aware of...' should be replaced by more concrete terms that link an activity to results or standards. It is helpful to state overall purposes and to categorise them into, say, clinical, managerial and educational sections. For example (managerial), 'To manage the service within the agreed budget.' If the task is to be done in conjunction with other staff, say so.

Personnel departments can help you to produce a job description (see page 145). They will have a standard pattern for job descriptions.

WHO IS WANTED?

Besides specifying the grade, key results, tasks and reporting arrangements for the job, you also need to identify the attributes that the post holder must have in order to succeed. This is known as the person specification.

Traditionally, the person specification is produced after the job description is drawn up. However, deriving one from the other, it is by no means an obvious or simple process. It is certainly not something to be left to the minute before the first candidate is interviewed. Note that the job description is not normally a list of candidate requirements or competencies, and it is unwise to treat it as such.

It is common for requirements to be specified in very broad terms using a checklist like Alec Rodger's famous seven-point plan, or the Munro Fraser five-point plan.

Rodger's seven-point plan asks you to consider requirements under the following headings:

- physique
- attainments
- intelligence
- aptitudes
- interests
- disposition
- circumstances.

Some people add motivation to the list. To use it, you simply specify your essential and desirable requirements under each heading. It is a simple, well-known and widely used checklist for deriving the person specification, but could be criticised on two counts. Firstly, it encourages too vague a definition of requirements, rather than sharply focusing on competencies. Secondly, several of the headings (like physique and circumstances) may lead to a too narrow definition of the *person* required for the job, and possibly in a way that discriminates against women or ethnic minorities, or creates a stereotype.

Drawing up this kind of person specification is a cumbersome process, which involves translating job tasks into general attributes thought necessary to do the job, assessing these for each candidate, and then predicting performance in specific areas on the basis of this assessment.

A more modern approach is to clearly specify competencies required and then to look for evidence of those same competencies. As a light-hearted example, I ask you to consider what makes a good clown, by clearly specifying competencies.

Example

Imagine that extensive research has revealed that a good performer will (say) consistently make children laugh, have a wide repertoire of tricks, and be able to perform to a high acrobatic

---

standard. A bad one will lack these qualities. We want these requirements to be our criteria for employing clowns. We also note that those clowns who fail to turn up on time for their performances cause problems, but this is not specific to the ability to perform the job of a clown, and is thus not part of our assessment of competence.

Competency 1: To be able to make children laugh

Here, it is hard to set standards, but we shall require evidence of the competency of clowns employed, or the circus could be in serious trouble.

Competency 2: To have a wide repertoire of acrobatic tricks

What, then, is a wide repertoire of tricks? We had better define a standard here. Let us say more than twenty.

If we want a high acrobatic standard, we may not actually want a specialist acrobat whose interests are more on perfecting high wire technique, and who will soon get bored with clowning. We could define it by specifying the kinds of exercises that we would want our clown to be able to do, to a given standard.

There is a common tendency to set qualification levels and experience requirements at too high a level. Even if you attract and recruit high calibre people, they may not be what you want. Moreover, you must always ask whether you can meet their high expectations.

Competency 3: To be able to ride a monocyle

This is a specific competency. I use the term 'competence' to describe the total ability to do the job. Normally, this involves a number of identifiable 'competencies' or specific abilities.

Have we now got the person specification we require for the clown job? It may define competence, but is that all we need? How can we be sure that our competent clown will also arrive on time? Might she be temperamental sometimes and refuse to perform?

Competencies tell you what the person 'can do', not what they 'will do'. Hence, there is also a need to consider the latter in some detail as well. These will be referred to as 'commitment' requirements. The competent employee may also be no more than adequate – you might be seeking the exceptional person. Here is a method that will help you.

Deriving a person specification from competence and commitment requirements (CCR method)

This section describes a method for deriving a person specification that covers both the 'can do' and 'will do' factors, which will be called competence and commitment, respectively.

Competence requirements

You are interested in finding out what the candidate 'can do' here. Potentially, this is an enormous list, so you will need to prioritise. It is usual to make assumptions very basic competencies, based on the candidate's work record or education. Those that are crucial to effectiveness in the job must be identified. These are the requirements that you must select especially for.

What kinds of competence? It may be in any of the following areas:

- clinical
- managerial
- general
- specialist.

Nursing competencies are defined statutorily, and these can be related to the job task, which provides a basic checklist (see page 132). You may also find the Whitley nurse clinical grading criteria useful here. Are you looking for a higher level than the basic statutory level? Certainly you are, if the person has to teach or manage others directly.

Management competencies are currently the source of much debate. There is probably no list of competencies that applies to all levels and all managerial jobs. The following checklist gives some guidance on the dimensions you should be looking at.

Checklist 16.1

1   Management task:
   - What will the person manage?
   - Project
   - Department
   - Activity, or technical or advisory service

- Change

  Each of these calls for slightly different competencies in managers.

2 Managing people:
- Self?
- Small team?
- Large team?
- Other managers?

  There are considerations here of level of authority, span of control and management style. Self-management will involve the ability to organise time and handle stress, for example.

3 Maintenance or innovation:
- Are you looking for strengths in fire-fighting or strategic planning?
- For short- or long-term problem solving?

4 Clarity and agreement on management task:
- How structured is the management task?
- Are the objectives clear?
- Are there diverse things or groups to co-ordinate or influence?
- Are prioritising and time management likely to be critical?
- Do you need a good negotiator? Or a creative policy maker?

5 People skills:
- Is there a premium on selecting, motivating, developing, correcting or counselling staff?
- What are the interpersonally sensitive issues the person will require skills to cope with?
- Will the person need a management style that emphasises leadership and control – or one that is able to reduce stress?

6 Analytical abilities:
- Are they likely to be important? You might need someone who is a sound analytical thinker, who can identify the right priorities.
- What skills in collecting or interpreting information are likely to be needed?

7 Communication skills:
- What kind of communication demands will there be? There will be a need to communicate effectively with the staff team. What about communication with senior management, outside bodies and other professionals?
- Are highly developed oral or written presentation skills essential?

General competencies should be identified for each kind of job in answer to the question: What other skills and knowledge are needed to carry out the job well? Typically, you might be looking for clear verbal expression, specific skills with people, ability to organise work, etc. The checklist for candidates might be useful here (see page 20).

If you require a high degree of technical expertise or skill, identify it under specialist competencies.

WARNINGS

1 Beware of identifying only vague abstractions, like 'must be a good leader'. It is better to say that the person requires the ability to maintain morale in a ward team under pressure, if that is what you really want.

2 Beware of creating too long a shopping list. You need to identify priorities. Pick only those competencies that seem to be critical for success – or where the person must be particularly strong.

3 Beware of looking for perfection. You will not find it, of course. You are often wise to avoid specifying a high-flier, if that is really not what you want, or what you will realistically recruit.

4 Anticipate the limitations of your selection techniques in getting evidence. You may not be able to assess specialised skills unless you see the person practicing. What the person says she can do may be all you can discover in some cases.

138

Commitment

We can define commitment as the factors that ensure that a person's abilities are used to the full for the benefit of the organisation. Here, we are concerned not so much with what the candidate 'can do' but rather what the candidate 'will do' if offered the post. All employers want commitment in their staff, but there is a danger of the interviewer interpreting commitment to mean 'the qualities that I have myself'.

Rather than use jargon words, like 'motivation', here, I prefer to use simple headings to identify different useful aspects:

- interests
- compatibility
- confidence
- application
- circumstances.

Interest requirements

What interests does the person need to have in order to find the work rewarding? Does a person's interests suggest that she will have a continued commitment? The interests may be in the technical aspects of the work, or in the social aspects. For instance, you may feel that work with children or elderly people requires evidence of a special interest. Someone might tell you she is a good manager, with no special interest in this field. Does that rule her out of the running? You might find that varied interests are necessary for some posts, while others may demand more single-track interests.

WARNINGS

Do not define interests too narrowly or make too much of them – interviewers often assume that candidates' interests have to match their own. If you are thinking of making certain interests a requirement, you have to challenge any assumptions you may be making first.

Compatibility requirements

In what respects must the person operate in ways compatible with others, and that of the section? Are her ideas compatible with the prevailing philosophy? Are there aspects of the person's personality that might be advantageous or disadvantageous? Will there need to be complete meshing with colleagues or other professionals? R M Belbin has identified the need to select people who perform complementary team roles – for example, an evaluator may be needed to complement an 'ideas person'. The person who is strong on initiation may need someone to finish the job.

WARNINGS

1 If you are not careful, you might select people who are clones of those already there. What may be good for the department is someone with different ideas; who is younger, or older; or who will challenge your cherished ideas; or who will play a role that is absent.

2 There is a danger of relying on your stereotypes and ignoring fresh qualities, although sometimes the opposite happens. A 'new broom' is chosen, who fails to achieve because the prevailing culture is alien. If you are going to talk about 'fitting in' – although I do not recommend it – it is essential that you know what sort of compatibility you want, and why. If the requirement has an adverse impact on one sex or ethnic group, you will be discriminating unfairly where the justifications of your requirements are in any way dubious (see page 166).

Confidence requirements

The standard question you will want to ask of all candidates will be: Does this person inspire confidence? You need to be sure that the otherwise competent person will actually do what you want her to. She must be manageable. That does not necessarily mean compliant. The basis of her co-operation with you may be having sufficient initiative to perform without having her hand held all of the time.

You do not want the kind of person who will be 'a law unto herself'. You may want the candidate to have a level of confidence in her own abilities, or some self-awareness, particularly of her style and the effect it has on others. Does she know her strengths and weaknesses, her limitations? She needs confidence in herself, and you need it in her.

Application requirements

Is there a crucial need to persist with all of the work objectives until they are achieved? In a demanding job, it may emphasise sheer energy, or determination. Perhaps the person has to overcome the negative attitudes of others. Perhaps the person needs to be resourceful and adaptable in pursuit of her goals. There may be a danger of a highly achieving individual pursuing her own personal goals to the detriment of those of the organisation. This is quite common in some teaching posts, for instance, where staff have a lot of freedom from supervision. Someone else may concentrate on what she is good at alone, or on just what is noticed and praised by others.

You may specify that you want someone with a track record of achievement – a cliché in management jobs. You may require that the person has the potential for promotion. This is a common requirement, but rather difficult to get sound evidence of – you would need to predict the person's future ability level as well as her ambition.

WARNINGS

One NHS employer who made previous regular progression in one's career a selection requirement found himself in an industrial tribunal, and indirect discrimination was proved against him. Lack of progression may have been because of previous unfair racial or sexual discrimination, so the requirement was potentially unfair to some candidates.

Circumstance requirements

Typically, you might want someone who is mobile, or capable of working irregular hours, or prepared to live near the job. More generally, you may want to ensure that there is nothing in the person's life that would interfere with regular attendance, limit her performance or force her to leave the post prematurely.

WARNINGS

Despite many warnings about asking women (but not men) about the demands their children would make, the practice persists. Here are three good reasons for avoiding it:

1   There is clearly an assumption that there will be a problem. This implies a requirement not to have dependent children,

which, even if asked of both sexes, indirectly discriminates against women, and cannot be justified as necessary for the job (see Chapter 19).

2 In practice, it is asked of women only, and this smacks of direct discrimination in thin disguise. The word will get around about this.

3 Many candidates will find it rather insulting that interviewers think that they are presenting themselves for employment without having thought out how they can cope with childminding commitments. Even if there was a problem, a candidate would be hardly likely to admit it.

If you impose unjustifiable requirements, like 'must be a single person', you unnecessarily limit your field, as well as risk infringing the law.

You can enter your requirements, along with details and standards, as your selection criteria on the recommended interview form (see Appendix 1). The following example shows one completed for the clown job. The right-hand side of the form is for recording evidence.

Example			
Name of candidate:		*Post*: Clown (grade 2)	
Criteria ::::::::::::::::::::::::::::::::		*Assessment* :::::::::::::::::::::::::::	
Requirements	Details and standards	Evidence found	Rating
Competencies	1 Able to make children laugh 2 Acrobatic competence on 20 standard tricks 3 Competent monocyclist		
Commitment Interests	1 Interest in children desirable		

142

	2	
Compatibility	Must adapt to fast pace of this circus quickly	
	3	
Confidence	Must work to directions from chief clown, have reliable timekeeping and personal behaviour	
	4	
Application	Previous star billing desirable	
	5	
Circumstances	Able to be away on tour regularly	

Other important considerations

Ready for the job right now – or growing into it?

You will need to consider whether a person will be able to grow into the job. The support and training available will be important here.

Do not idealise

Avoid creating a picture of an ideal person, who probably doesn't exist, or locking your mind into the idea of one type of person, particularly if it resembles the person who is leaving the job. Think of as many different ways of doing the job as possible.

Reflect on and test your ideas about what is required

Imagine, for instance, how you might handle the tricky parts of the job and how colleagues might do it differently. You need to be able to identify the characteristics that would rule people out, and the essential positive qualities that are needed. Test these out with colleagues, to check that you are not seeing the job too narrowly, or in terms of particular stereotypes.

The following checklist summarises the steps involved in preparing a person specification.

SHARPENING CRITERIA

Essentials and desirables

One way of sharpening criteria is to distinguish essential requirements from those that are merely desirable. Where the minimal requirement for a post in an elderly care unit might be several years of experience of elderly care in a number of settings, having undertaken an ENB course on the care of the elderly might be seen as a desirable extra, but not essential.

Critical attributes for success

One promising new approach uses people's past knowledge of the post in question to identify important qualities – these are the things that are found to distinguish good practitioners from bad ones, most usefully described in terms of competencies (Janz).

You can find these critical attributes through your own research, typically by systematic comparison of past good performers and bad ones on a number of dimensions of performance, or by examining critical incidents that have been the 'make-or-break' factors in the eyes of good practitioners and their bosses.

It is important to discover what the key attributes are and then to design your assessment procedures, to discover whether candidates possess these attributes. We will look at this again in Chapter 17.

USING THE PERSONNEL OFFICER

Do not neglect the people whose job it is to help you to select. You will find that they bring realism into your visions. They may comment on the job description ('This is far too much for one job') or the person specification ('You won't find this person on this earth'). From their knowledge of the job market, they can give advice on how to attract the right candidate. They might suggest that you introduce flexibility, novel recruitment methods ('This would be a good post for job share') and so on. The following checklist indicates what areas to discuss with personnel officers.

Checklist 16.3

1 The general recruitment and selection policies.
2 About the vacancy:
   ● Could the job description be improved?
   ● Is the grade and skill level appropriate?
   ● Is your person specification realistic?
   ● Could the hours be different, part-time, more flexible?
   ● Are there possible internal candidates?
3 About publicising the vacancy:
   ● What could be an inducement for people to apply?
   ● How should the job be promoted and advertised?
   ● How long will it take?
   ● What should the advertisement look like?
   ● How much will it cost?
   ● What kind of response can be expected?
   ● What recruitment procedure is recommended?
   ● What is other people's experience in advertising for similar posts?
   ● Are you observing equal opportunities requirements?
4 About the recruitment process in the organisation:
   ● What are the standard procedures for recruitment, advertising and interviewing?

- Who should be doing what, and when?
- What professional support can the personnel officer provide you with?
- What budget can you call on?
- What facilities are available for marketing the post? (For example, publicity material, expert help in drafting copy, or involvement in careers conventions or job forums?)
- Where can the interview take place?
- Is an assessor required, and can one be found?
- Will the personnel department arrange for references to be taken up?
- Can the personnel department arrange for health checks to be carried out?
- Or, if appropriate:
  For any kind of testing to be done on candidates?
  To attend the interview?
  To arrange tours of the site?
  To give details of the post and terms and conditions to enquirers — in person or by telephone?

REFERENCES

Belbin, R M, *Management Teams: Why They Succeed or Fail* (Heinemann, 1981).

Fraser, John Munro, *Employment Interviewing*, 5th Edn (MacDonald and Evans, 1978).

Janz, T, Hellervik, L and Gilmore, D, *Behaviour Description Interviewing* (Allyn & Bacon, 1986).

Rodger, Alec, *The Seven Point Plan*, 3rd Edn (National Institute of Industrial Psychology, 1970).

FURTHER READING

Rawling, Ken, *The Seven Point Plan and New Perspectives Fifty Years on* (NFER – Nelson, 1985).

Ungerson, B, *How to Write a Job Description* (IPM, 1983).

Chapter 17

SELECTION STRATEGY

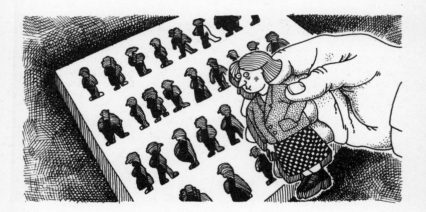

CHOOSING A SELECTION DEVICE

Having defined what you want, how do you find out if the candidates have it? There are a number of selection devices available, of which the interview is only one, and it may not be the best.

You could assess the person's competence in a number of ways. You will remember the clown in the last chapter who was required to make children laugh, perform acrobatic tricks and ride the monocycle. How might he (or should I say she) be assessed? The following example describes some possibilities.

Example

1 Ability test:
   Here is a monocycle. Can you ride it across the room please?

2 Psychometric assessment:
   Your results on this pencil and paper test show that you are likely to relate well to children.

3 Hypothetical questions:
   Imagine you see a child crying in the street. Tell me how you could make her laugh?

4 Test or sample knowledge:
   What is the best way to keep your balance on a wire?

Instead of sampling the person's competence directly, here and now, you might explore her past record instead, as best you can.

5 Biographical data:
   She is the eldest of a large family. She will have had to amuse the younger ones.

6 References:
   The ringmaster says she had dozens of superb tricks.

7 Interview discussion and judgement:
   You probed deeply and concluded that she really does know how to make children laugh.

8 Self-report:
   She described herself as a very good clown.

9 Documented evidence:
   She showed me certificates for acrobatic achievement and a videotape of her in action.

As this example shows, you sometimes have to rely on the candidate's word. However, you are able to get better evidence by using more than one device. You can use this to corroborate evidence.

When you are looking for particular requirements, you need to gear your method to the assessment of those qualities – the videotape or demonstration of acrobatic qualities would be better than some written report. In general, the more sampling of actual behaviour (as opposed to a report) you can do, the better; and the greater the number of different assessments you do, the more accurate the overall assessment decision is likely to be.

No assessment or test criterion you use can ever be perfect. You may label as bad, some people who would in practice be good; conversely, you may label as good, some who turn out in practice to be bad. If you are concerned about not missing any possibly good people, you can lower your 'pass mark' on the test, but you are then bound to let more bad candidates through. On the other hand, if you are concerned with finding only the best, then you raise the 'pass mark', and eliminate some who would have succeeded in practice.

There is usually a need for some initial screening or shortlisting, but you need to be selective in what you read into application forms and CVs. There is no harm in asking candidates to answer specific sections related to the requirements of a particular job. This enhances the capacity to distinguish suitable from unsuitable applicants, whereas using an unreliable criterion like 'good handwriting' merely reduces the field of applicants.

References need to be used. They can be structured to reveal specific information that is related to the criteria you have set. We discuss the use of references in more detail in Chapter 20.

APPLICATION FORMS

Many organisations ask for a curriculum vitae these days. This cuts out one stage in the recruitment process, and saves on postage, but it often means that the information the recruiter might especially want is missing. Each CV will be in a different form.

If you want the candidate to think hard about the job before applying, it will be better to send an application form out with the recruitment package. Make sure that the sections on any application form are all relevant to the job being applied for. Leave specific health questions out of the application form. It is sometimes useful to ask candidates for additional information. Where recently qualified staff are being recruited, it will often be of interest to see where their interests lie, or how they write about themselves and their ideas. Such extra questions should require only brief answers. If the standard application form is off-putting, seek to design your own.

There is no reason at all why you should not supplement your application form with additional questions that are relevant, and that will help you to shortlist. The standard application form asks people to give additional material in support of their application. You can, instead, ask for an essay or a report on a particular subject. You could ask for relevant factual details, or for their opinions. I have found it useful to ask people to make lists of reasons why they want to work in a particular field (to test their specific motivation), or to give their views on some current developments (to test their awareness, or capacity to do some research). You may get some idea of their analytical or written communication skills from their replies – but be wary of setting too much store by this. The following example gives a sample of additional questions that could be added to an application form in particular cases.

Example

1 For post of community services manager:
   In 50 words or less, say what you think will be the impact of Project 2000 on the nursing services in the community. List up to six issues in order of priority.

2 For specialised clinical work:
   What do you feel are your main strengths in relation to this job? Are there areas where you feel you would need further training or support?

3 For a clinical researcher:
   Please give a summary (40 words) of some research you have carried out recently. Explain how you came to do this piece of research, and your choice of methodology.

On the whole, people prefer to be tested in this way, rather than to be put on the spot in the interview. You will have excellent material to probe further at the interview – and that process tends to sort out those who have copied out an answer without having understood it.

HIGHER HURDLES?

Can you improve selection simply by making the hurdles higher – by setting higher standards? Yes, if you are sure the hurdles are suitable ones in the first place. But if they are not, then making them higher will result in more good applicants being eliminated, as well as bad. So if you think that very neat handwriting is an indicator of being 'well-organised', and you shortlist people on this basis, then you will eliminate all the well-organised people whose handwriting happens to be less than very neat.

FINDING BETTER SIGNALS OF FUTURE SUCCESS

It might be useful, then, to look at just *what* you are taking to be signals of future success. What actually correlates with success or with particular desirable qualities? If you can devise a system for scoring individuals on factors that you know from past experience to correlate with future success, you can use the scoring system to predict others who are likely to succeed (assuming you are agreed on what constitutes success!). For instance, you may discover from your research that people who have chopped and changed jobs in the past are likely to do so in the future. If scored in some way, this is the basis of a useful predictor. This method of detecting the best signals is called Biodata, and can be applied to the selection of learners. It improves your use of information about the past, which predicts how people will behave in the future.

In using it, you must be sure that you are not merely detecting factors that reflect privileges that have allowed people access to success in the past.

NOT SAYING BUT DOING

You may be too much influenced by what people say they can do. To find out how they actually perform, why not simulate parts of the job? Candidates could be asked to make presentations, to write reports, to undertake 'in tray' exercises, or to take part in discussions on group tasks. You could ask someone to demonstrate a clinical procedure she said she knew about. This is known as work sampling.

Simply jumping into a role play in the middle of the interview will not do, however. You will need to plan the exercise, and it should be realistic. You should test the rating scale (and your raters) beforehand, if you want fairness and consistency. What is being assessed must be relevant to the job. Where the effort and cost is seen to be worthwhile, several performance assessments may be combined in a so-called assessment centre. This was described in Chapter 10.

A further available method is psychometric assessment,

usually reserved for senior appointments. We looked at this briefly in Chapter 10.

Instead of interviewing candidates, perhaps you could simply put them all in a room with a pencil and paper and get them to do a number of tests. A psychologist might then tell you all about each candidate, and who to select. The job would be done for you, and many psychologists would say it would be done more accurately. Few would find this strategy acceptable though.

Table 17.1 gives a summary of the kinds of psychometric assessments available.

Table 17.1 *Types of psychometric test*

Test	Indications
General ability tests	Measure ability to reason, using words, numbers or abstract material. They can be set at different levels: correct and incorrect responses. High reliability and validity.
Specific ability and aptitude tests	Measure particular skills and aptitudes – for example, computer aptitude, word fluency, manual dexterity, typing speed. Generally reliable.
Personality assessments	Measure traits or personal styles. No 'correct' answers. Lower validity and reliability.

These cost around £600 per person by outside consultants. You can be trained to administer some yourself, particularly ability tests, which tend to be cheaper and have higher validities.

The following checklist summarises the selection options open to interviewers.

Checklist 17.1

1 Sample current performance (work sampling) or assess past record (Biodata).
2 Data from candidate alone (CV) or data from other sources (references).
3 Highly specific factors (ability test) or broad-range factors (application form).

---

4 Known validity and reliability (personality inventory) or unknown validity and reliability (references and interview).

5 Selection standards set low (more false positives – suitable for preliminary screening) or high (more false negatives – suitable for final selection).

FURTHER READING

Anastasi, A, *Psychological Testing*, 5th Edn (Collier Macmillan, 1988).

Bayne, R, *et al.*, 'Board and selection interviews in selection: an experimental study of their comparative effectiveness', *Personnel Review*, **12**(3), 1983.

Bolton, G M, *Interviewing for Selection Decisions* (NFER – Nelson, 1983).

Buckingham, G, 'Using structured interviews to measure job success', *Personnel Management*, **17**(10), 1985.

Cook, Mark, *Personnel Selection and Productivity* (Wiley, 1988).

Courtis, J, *The IPM Guide to Cost Effective Recruitment*, 2nd Edn (IPM, 1985).

Drenth, P, 'Principles of selection', in *Psychology at Work*, 2nd Edn, Warr, Ed (Penguin Education, 1978).

Dulewicz, V, 'Assessment centres as the route to competence', *Personnel Management*, November 1989.

IPM Code on Occupational Testing (IPM, 1989).

Jeffrey, R, 'Taking the guesswork out of selection', *Personnel Management*, **9**(10), 1977.

Lewis, C, 'What's new in selection', *Personnel Management*, **16**(1), 1984.

Makin, P and Robertson, I, 'Selecting the best selection techniques', *Personnel Management*, **18**(11), 1986.

Palmer, R, 'A sharper focus for the panel interview', *Personnel Management*, **15**(5), 1983.

Psychological Testing (Personnel Management, Factsheet No. 24, 1989).

Pursell, E D, *et al.*, 'Structured interviewing: avoiding selection problems', *Personnel Journal*, **59**(11), 1980.

Robertson, Ivan and Iles, Paul, 'Approaches to managerial selection', in *International Review of Industrial and Organisational Psychology*, I Cooper and I Robertson, Eds (Wiley, 1988).

Smith, M, Gregg, M and Andrews, D, *Selection and Assessment* (Pitman, 1989).

Smith, M and Robertson, I T, *The Theory and Practice of Systematic Staff Selection* (Macmillan, 1986).

Toplis, J, Dulewicz, V and Fletcher, C, *Psychological Testing: A Practical Guide* (IPM, 1987).

Tyler, Leona E, *Tests and Measurements*, 3rd Edn (Prentice-Hall International, 1979).

Chapter 18

THE RECRUITMENT SELECTION PROCESS OVERALL

It is time to look at the necessary administrative support that is involved in recruitment and selection. Much of this will be in the hands of the personnel department.

As a manager wanting to select staff, it is important that you understand the processes involved thoroughly. Flowchart B, on page 113, gives an overview of the whole recruitment selection process. In later chapters, we will cover important aspects like advertising, shortlisting and the taking up of references in detail, before we discuss the interview itself.

THE ESSENTIALS

Five things are essential in any recruitment process. We shall bear these in mind as we look at the management of the important stages between the placing of the advertisement and the interview.

Effective communication

In the early stages of recruitment, you will be concerned with getting a message over to all those who may be interested. Later, you will be concerned about gaining trust and commitment. Recruiting is like performing a play. All those involved must know their parts. There must be good communication between them. All documents must support the message and style. Misconceptions lead to expensive mistakes.

Speed of response

Often, there is an urgency in filling the post. Even if there is not, too much delay will mean losing good candidates, who are being sought by others and will not wait for you. So you need to ensure that you are quick off the mark and at the same time thorough.

Consideration to candidates

This should include the need to be fair and to comply with legal requirements. The important issue of equal opportunities is covered in Chapter 19.

It will also mean being as helpful and informative as possible, and being aware of what is important to candidates – especially their time, trouble and desire not to be embarrassed or harassed. How can this be built into the recruitment process?

Often, one hears that the date of an interview, which took an interminably long time to set up, has been sent to candidates with three days' notice, giving them a real problem in getting time off to attend. In one such interview, candidates were nevertheless expected to decide whether to accept an offer on the spot.

Effective matching

Obviously, you want to find the right people. This may be easy, where your criteria are straightforward, easily assessable and not too critical – 'desirable' rather than 'essential' requirements. Often, however, the criteria are none too clear, and none too easy to assess. What is more, the consequences of failure may sometimes be painful, expensive and protracted. Matching must also involve meeting the candidates' requirements, including, for instance, somewhere to live.

Some of the matching process will be concerned with screening out unsuitable people. But you need to know what the limits are. Over-elaborate selection will take time and could be inconsiderate to candidates. It may be appropriate sometimes to recruit the first person who meets the criteria; in others, you are well advised to recruit the best you can find.

The need to be flexible

Different recruitment situations dictate different degrees of priority. Sometimes speed will be crucial, sometimes precision of assessment. However, there needs to be a balance between them. Over-emphasis on one can damage the others.

A manager had a job that was proving hard to fill. She was impatient with the results from the personnel department. She met a man in a pub on holiday and there and then offered him the job. He seemed to have the right skills, and he was interested. He later telephoned the personnel department, informing them that his house was on the market, and that he was waiting to join. He found that the salary on offer was not what the manager had offered. He had also been told that his removal expenses would be paid, but the personnel department said that this was not the case.

Getting this process right requires a clear idea of what is required, and a clear idea of who has to do what to make it happen. The latter puts a premium on good planning and briefing of people, so they know what is expected of them.

KEY STAGES

The matching process will involve a set series of stages, which are described in flowchart B, on page 113, including:

1   A decision to fill the vacancy.

2   Identification of the requirements.

3   Creation of the person specification and selection criteria. These issues were covered in Chapter 16.

4   Decisions on selection methods. Chapters 15 and 17 described what is available.

5   The advertisement. This is the trigger to the response. It sets the tone and the time fuse.

6   Sending out the information pack and application form. This is discussed from the candidate's point of view in Chapter 3, and from the employer's in Chapter 19. It is a good idea to see it from the candidate's point of view. A good information pack is essential these days if you are to have any hope of attracting staff from outside.

7   The response to enquiries. The first human contact needs to be positive, friendly and well-informed. It is best if it is from the manager in person.

8   Various stages of screening (by both employer and prospective candidate). Candidates need to know what sort of race they are being invited to compete in. Encourage them until you or they can decide that there is a mismatch. The employer will want a manageable but adequate interview shortlist of candidates, and all candidates should appear appointable on paper.

   Health screening and references will also be needed.

   Candidates' criteria must be part of the agenda, too. Not least of these is salary and accommodation.

9   Assessment of candidates (and of job). The processes must be fair (all through) and must clearly identify those people who meet the criteria set. Processes must be efficient and reliable – you do not want to reject good people.

10   Offer and negotiation. The wanted fish must be landed. Others must not be discouraged.

11   Offers of feedback to candidates. We discuss this in Chapter 25. This should be considered an important, if tricky, part of good practice.

12   Follow through and evaluation. Many people think that it all ends when the candidate accepts. But there is a need to ensure that details are transmitted for induction, that the whole process is reviewed to identify improvements, and that the criteria and selection judgements are validated. In practice, this scarcely happens.

ADMINISTRATION

Administration should be invisible. Every link in the flowchart is important. A number of departments will be involved. Attention to detail is important. Will there be enough room in the car park? Will the coffee arrive on time? Will the receptionist know where to send the candidate who arrives at the wrong hospital? Can the clerk who processes the applications be relied upon to be efficient and follow the equal opportunities policy to the letter? Will the panel keep to time?

However good your ideas on recruitment and selection, if the impression given is that of an administrative shambles, you will never get the people you want. Word soon gets around that you are not worth bothering with.

THE TREND TO COMPLICATION

The whole process can become long, drawn out and complicated for a number of reasons. More stages come to be built in to ensure that the right things are done by the right people, and that everything is seen to be fair. In attempting to meet equal opportunities requirements, attention has rightly been drawn to sources of bias in procedures. The response has often been to make them more complicated and more formal, and sometimes to suggest to line managers that they cannot be trusted to make decisions on their own. Alternatively, managers could be made accountable, and made aware of the issues through better training.

As other organisations find clever and legally acceptable ways of cutting corners, we are in danger of creating in the NHS the most bureaucratic recruitment procedures in Europe. The following procedure is typical.

An advertisement is placed with a closing date. Often, there is an 'internal trawl' for candidates, followed by public advertising. Candidates are invited to write for an application form. They are sent one, possibly without any further information about the job. These application forms are received, and certain individuals are shortlisted and invited for interview on a certain date, usually not negotiable. By this time, some two months have passed. References are taken up.

The candidates come for interview. They stay all day and wait hours to be called for a 45-minute conversation with a panel, none of whom they will meet before, nor afterwards.

A week later, sometimes two, an offer is made to one candidate. When, and only when, she has put her acceptance in writing, the other candidates are sent curt 'regret' letters from the personnel department telling them that they have been unsuccessful (but not why). No feedback on their interview performance is offered.

At each of these stages, it is easy to imagine candidates withdrawing. Some will have found it all too tedious; others will have found other jobs; others will have been unable to attend the interview.

Contrast this with the practice of some commercial employers. They will advertise a post (sometimes without a closing date). The manager concerned will welcome telephone calls from all those interested. Long conversations with enquirers will ensue, where the possibilities of a match between person and job are explored. An invitation to make an informal visit may be offered. Frequently, a job interview will also be arranged at a time to suit the individual. The full recruitment package will be sent out, and only then will a full CV or application form be asked for. CVs are sometimes sought early on and used as the basis for the informal discussion with the enquirer.

Outside the public services, references are only normally requested when an offer is made.

This 'fast uptake' system does in fact operate in the NHS, particularly when seeking staff nurses in unpopular specialties. What are the pros and cons?

Communication is direct, cutting out clerks and personnel assistants. Consequently, the manager has to know what she can offer. But the manager is also free to discriminate unfairly, and if she chooses to 'fob off' people she does not like, she is not normally monitored in this. The candidate who is offered the interview will perceive a personalised interest in her. The response is also impressively fast.

If you know you have several vacancies to be filled urgently, you may be able to make some offers without seeing the whole field. Otherwise, there will be a need to consider all of the candidates who apply before you can make any offer. You could get a lot of interest from suitable candidates and find yourself obliged to see all of them.

All the same, you could well encourage such early discussions. You could establish a useful early rapport and build on it during the informal visit. Greater flexibility in interviewing practices is also needed, although admittedly this is difficult for senior appointments where large hard-to-convene panels are the norm.

A salutary experience is losing catering staff to a rival who is able to interview and offer jobs all on the same morning that the candidates made their enquiry. This forced me to introduce a similar system, with a helpful occupational health department providing an 'on call' service. I also worked with a DNS colleague to ensure that we could always offer interviews to staff nurses within a day or two of enquiry, using a rota of senior nurses, linked to OHD. The job offers were not far behind – there are obvious dangers in rushing candidates.

If you are recruiting, you should have an 'on call' service to enquirers. A good secretary is not enough. The recruiting manager or a close associate who has been well briefed to pick up the enquiry or show people around should be available in person.

The complete procedure, including dates and times, should be drawn up well in advance and be available to everyone involved, including temporary secretaries and post clerks. They will be briefed to spot a coded vacancy number on an envelope, which signifies an application, and know what to do with it. Everything that happens, each respondent, each call and each decision (with reasons) has to be recorded. Plan to be flexible but organised. Do not allow long chains or bottlenecks.

Reply personally, confirm conversations in writing and show urgency, but give adequate lead-in time and response time. Explain delays. Do not leave people 'hanging on'. Your personnel officer will be your guide in all of these areas (see Chapter 16).

FURTHER READING

Courtis, J, *The IPM Guide to Cost Effective Recruitment*, 2nd Edn (IPM, 1985).

Croner's Guide to Interviews (Croner, 1985).

Equal Opportunities Commission, *Fair and Efficient Selection: Guidance on Equal Opportunities Policies in Recruitment and Selection Procedures* (EOC, 1986).

IDS, *Race and Sex Discrimination: Recruitment Arrangements* (IDS, Brief No. 324, 1986).

Interviewing within the law, *Employment Digest*, **239**, 1988.

IPM Equal Opportunities Code (Institute of Personnel Management, 1989).

IPM Recruitment Code (Institute of Personnel Management, 1989).

Jessup, Gilbert and Jessup, Helen, *Selection and Assessment at Work* (Methuen, 1975).

Personnel & Training Management Yearbook and Directories (Kogan Page).

Plumbley, P, *Recruitment and Selection*, 4th Edn (IPM, 1985).

Shouksmith, George, *Assessment through Interviewing* (Pergamon Press, 1978).

Sidney, E, *Managing Recruitment* (Gower, 1988).

Ungerson, B, Ed, *Recruitment Handbook*, 3rd Edn (Gower, 1988).

Chapter 19

ADVERTISING THE JOB

THE ADVERTISEMENT ITSELF

Find an original angle when you are designing an advertisement. Stress what is special and the unique selling points. See it from the candidates' viewpoint. Arouse their curiosity, interest and admiration. Write in a clear style with no redundant words. Avoid phoniness and clichés. Do not oversell. Personalise where necessary. Check details, including spelling and grammar. Remember the press deadlines, and make sure you are ready to respond to applicants in a speedy and friendly way. The following example highlights the selling features of an advertisement.

Example

Nursing Press requires advertising copy (top grade)

- Are you the advertisement we are looking for?
- Do you attract attention?
- Can you convey the essence of the job and the organisation?
- Can you describe the important qualities needed in a way that people can start to match themselves to?

If so, we can promise you a successful career in our successful magazine. You will be lively and memorable. Contact us personally by the closing date. We are non-smokers and believe in equal opportunities, progressive care and the power of the printed word.

It is noticeable in the NHS that, since their prohibition by the Rayner Scrutiny, display advertisements are creeping back, even

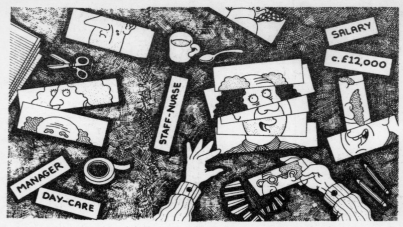

for non-managerial posts, with the trend being led by teaching and special health authorities. Your personnel officer will advise you on when to splash out on a display advertisement. It is more expensive, and in many cases it will not secure a competitive advantage.

The following checklist outlines the points to cover in an advertisement.

Checklist 19.1

1 Health authority title.
2 Unit title.
3 Location.
4 Job.
5 Grade.
6 Details of the unit or department.
7 Job details (salary scale optional).
8 What is offered (experience, training, accommodation).
9 Requirements (experience, qualifications, interests).
10 Contact for further information.
11 Contact for application form.
12 Closing date.
13 Policy on equal opportunities or smoking (optional).

Here are some real-life examples from the *Nursing Times*:

A vacancy has arisen for an enthusiastic and well-motivated person.

This is the standard, current cliché again. Its meaning is unclear. Who would want an unenthusiastic poorly motivated nurse?

Many advertisements say what the employers want from the candidates (ENB courses, etc.) without stressing what they can offer candidates. Try starting with what you can offer. Then, further down, state your requirements and restrict the field to those you want.

More interesting opening lines include:

Would you like to be part of the hospital's shop window? Would you like every weekend free? (OPD ad)

Associate nurse – grade E – for the elderly and casualty. This unusual and interesting combination gives nurses the opportunity to further their skills in both specialties.

Are you an experienced RGN looking for hours to suit your busy lifestyle? (G grade twilight community nurse)

Would you like to work in a patient-orientated, progressive, friendly and busy ophthalmic ward whose philosophy hopes to encompass 'primary nursing' by 1990?

On the other hand, how about:

There are now vacancies for staff nurses to join our team of staff maintaining 24-hour nursing cover within the elderly care services unit. The successful applicant will have a minimum of one year's post-registration experience and a general commitment to caring for elderly people. Apply to. . .

or:

RGN grade F required for theatres. Must have relevant experience.

or:

Staff nurse grade D required for genito-urinary department. Full- or part-time considered, minimum of 28 hours. Salary. . .

Small details can make or mar an advertisement. If a visit is offered, it is so much friendlier to ask people to ring a named person rather than someone called, for example, assistant director of nursing services (staff support). The effect of one very well constructed and friendly advertisement was jarred by the inclusion of 'Write to the personnel department in "H block" for a form'. Another opened 'We have a vacancy for an experienced and enthusiastic nurse to be block based'. Yet another advertisement offered '. . .positions in a team which saw 33,000 children last year'. The National Heart Hospital advertisement sets the scene with 'Just another day of quiet dramas. . . each day provides its continuing blend of pressures and satisfactions. . .'.

WHICH MEDIUM?

Your personnel department or advertising agency will advise you on this. They will probably tell you that local newspapers may be effective in attracting unqualified nurses but carry little advertising for qualified staff, and none at all for specialised professionals. This means that professional magazines like the *Nursing Times* are the best media to use for any professional post. You will not attract the people you want by advertising in the local paper if nurses never think of looking there for jobs.

Local papers with a wider regional circulation are sometimes used successfully for advertising managerial posts, and can sometimes be effective for attracting qualified nurses.

RECORD THE RESPONSE

It is important to check the response to every advertisement you use. You will be interested in how many people respond to each advertisement, how many apply for the job and how many turn out to be suitable. Careful analysis can point to the media, format and advertising schedules that give you the best results and value from your advertising budget.

To safeguard against any advertising becoming too selective and, therefore, possibly unfairly discriminatory, it is advisable to make details of all vacancies available to the local job centre.

Unless there is succession planning in your unit, you will probably want to advertise the post internally, but not necessarily externally, if there are likely to be good internal candidates. There may be an equal opportunities issue to consider here, if by so doing you are excluding some people from the opportunity to apply. You may need to bring in an outside assessor to judge whether any internal candidate will be up to the mark.

THE RECRUITMENT INFORMATION PACKAGE

It is important for staff who work in the department where the vacancy has arisen to be involved in recruitment. Ask them to write a brief 'patch profile' of the department's history, its location and what makes it tick. This should then be edited and included in the recruitment package for potential candidates.

Ask what is important to them, what they believe about patient care, and what they would like people to know about. Reflect history and talk about the importance of the location, and let them say why they are special.

Such an exercise is good for morale, and also relays to candidates that the place is being run by human beings, not robots. It can also give some colour to the advertisement, if you want it to.

The patch profile should be part of the information package for candidates, which should include the items listed in the following checklist.

Checklist 19.2

1 Job:
- Job description.
- Organisation charts.
- Details of job requirements (person specification).
- Details of the selection process, with relevant dates.
- Application form (if used), and how and to whom to apply.
2 Benefits and amenities:
- Details of remuneration.
- Other benefits of working in the district, including assistance with accommodation, transport and childminding, and details of local amenities, with a map.
3 Professional:
- Details of services and philosophy of care.
- The 'patch profile' and objectives of the unit.
- Opportunities for training and professional development.
- Many authorities include well-produced catalogues of all local post-basic and management training opportunities as well as relevant service reports.
- Covering letter with details of informal visits offered.

A personalised covering letter should thank people for their enquiry and remind them of the closing date. It should be friendly and enthusiastic, welcome the recipients to come for an informal visit and encourage them to apply.

Some employers will include the person specification, to indicate 'the kind of person we are looking for'. Some, on the other hand, still send nothing but the application form!

Even if the enquirers do not apply, they will be sufficiently impressed to consider applying for other posts in that authority, if the information package is interesting, professional and friendly.

The person specification will not only show that you have thought deeply about the kind of person you are looking for, it will also help the candidates to match their own profile to yours. If you think that revealing your requirements explicitly will give candidates an easy opportunity to present themselves as 'just what you are looking for', you should consider two things: whether you will be so easily fooled if the person is pretending; and also whether it helps you to have a lot of inappropriate applications that result from an ignorance of the requirements. Intelligent candidates will, in any case, make sure that they have a shrewd idea of your requirements when they apply.

EQUAL OPPORTUNITIES CONSIDERATIONS

One of your concerns in advertising will be to avoid any suggestion of unfair discrimination. This does not simply mean keeping out of legal trouble. It means presenting your organisation as fair in its practices, and offering genuine equality of opportunity. Let us start by examining discrimination, as defined in the Race Relations Act and the Sex Discrimination Act.

Direct discrimination is treating people less favourably on the grounds of their sex or race. Discrimination against married people is covered in the Sex Discrimination Act, while the Race Relations Act embraces discrimination on the grounds of colour, ethnic or national origins, or nationality.

Indirect discrimination is a more difficult concept. It occurs where a rule or requirement is applied to everyone but has an adverse impact on one sex or particular racial groups; where the rule or requirement cannot be justified as being necessary for the job. The adverse impact implies detriment or disadvantage, and a disproportionate effect between sexes or racial groups. How disproportionate does the effect have to be? Twenty per cent differences would suffice.

The rule or requirement will not be seen as necessary for the job when a less discriminatory one can be substituted for it with the same effect. What may be desirable has to be distinguished from what is actually a requirement for the job. A requirement for 'fluency in Asian languages' would be justifiable only if the job required communication with people who only spoke these languages. A requirement that 'mother tongue must be English' would be harder to justify, and would constitute indirect discrimination, but a requirement for 'fluency in English' would be a less discriminatory equivalent. This would have the same effect, and would be acceptable if a relevant requirement.

It is unlawful to publish advertisements that indicate or 'might reasonably be understood as indicating' an intention to discriminate on racial or sexual grounds. The test of this is what the average reader would take it to mean.

An advertisement for a ward sister, which did not specify that a charge nurse would also be acceptable, might be direct discrimination.

The following example gives further illustrations of unfair discrimination.

Example

1 In an advertisement, you ask for specific academic qualifications. This is indirect discrimination if significantly fewer women or people of ethnic minorities can comply, unless the qualification is essential and exclusive. Sometimes adding 'or equivalent standard' to your specified qualification may help.

2 A recruitment picture depicting workers who are all white males. This could be direct discrimination if the average reader might presume that women or non-white people are not welcome.

3 Recruitment from certain areas only. This has been proven to be indirect discrimination.

4 Recruitment by word of mouth only; recruitment by taking on people who write speculative letters of application. There is a good chance that you will be effectively excluding some groups who may not be aware of the contacts.

5 Judging facility for manual work from handwritten application screening. This is not justifiable. If it can be proven to have an adverse impact on ethnic minorities, it is indirect discrimination.

6 Giving preference regularly to people from certain training schools. This could well be indirect discrimination, and unlawful, since as a requirement it is unlikely to be justifiable.

7 Rejection of young married women on the grounds that they are more likely to become pregnant. This is likely to be direct discrimination.

8 Favouring people with particular hobbies or outside interests. Like all arbitrary criteria it is hard to justify in job terms, and could well be detrimental to certain groups. It is, therefore, possibly indirect discrimination.

---

9 Applying maximum age limits. It has been established in industrial tribunals that to discriminate against women and ethnic minorities in this way will constitute indirect discrimination.

10 Turning away or putting off people from particular ethnic backgrounds. This is direct discrimination.

11 No clear criteria set for selection; no written documentation of selection decisions. While this in itself would be hard to indict as discriminatory practice, the industrial tribunal may well regard it as evidence of poor practice, which may well conceal direct and indirect discrimination.

Some implications of discriminatory practices

The obvious one is that the organisation gets a bad name, and may be fined for transgressing the law. The practices also discourage and debar many suitable applicants from the ethnic minorities (or perhaps women), and limit the labour pool from which recruitment takes place. For some qualified staff, this pool is reducing anyway, so employers who engage in this practice are reducing further their chances of acquiring suitable staff.

Good practice

The Commission for Racial Equality (CRE) has published a Code of Practice. Failure to comply with this will be seen as an indicator that an organisation has scant regard for compliance with the discrimination law. Moreover, this, together with a study of equal opportunities policies in operation, will be taken into account when discrimination cases are heard against that employer, although failure to comply is not in itself unlawful.

In summary, it urges employers to have a meaningful equal opportunities policy. It strongly recommends the monitoring of all employment practices, especially those in recruitment. It asks employers to ensure that all 'gatekeepers' who give access to jobs or information are trained in equal opportunities practice, and understand their legal and social obligations. Criteria by which decisions are made should be explicit and of proven relevance. Selection methods should be open to scrutiny, and should be consistent. Employers should not take chances by allowing recruitment decisions to be in the hands of one person only, or by allowing informal recruitment, for instance by word of mouth alone. All judgements and decisions should be recorded, with reasons, and kept for inspection.

The CRE Code of Practice encourages employers to keep records of employees, including their ethnic origin, in order to monitor the performance of the policy in reaching targets. Thus, personnel departments may send out a form asking candidates to state their ethnic origin, explaining why this is wanted.

The practices of organisations are in fact very visible to outsiders. The concern for equality of opportunity makes a lot of sense if one is looking for high standards of recruitment and the best possible choice of staff.

REFERENCE

Commission for Racial Equality, *Code of Practice for the Elimination of Discrimination and the Promotion of Equality of Opportunity in Employment* (CRE, 1984).

FURTHER READING

IDS, *Race and Sex Discrimination: Recruitment Arrangements* (IDS, Brief No. 324, 1986).

Ray, M, *Recruitment Advertising: A Means of Communication* (IPM, 1980).

Chapter 20

PRELIMINARY SCREENING

Study the past if you would divine the future.   Confucius, *Analects*

DECIDING TO SHORTLIST

When the advertisement is placed, you will not know whether or not you will need to shortlist. It is wise to plan for it, and to identify your selection panel as the best people to do it. You will, at the very least, find a second opinion helpful, and despite the current general management ethos, you may want to encourage corporate ownership of the decision. If you go solo and show bias, you may be called to task for flouting equal opportunity policies, or upsetting the consultant whose support is vital.

You will not always want to shortlist – you may be seeing everybody, or nobody. It is in the latter case that the criteria derived from your person specification will be put to the test. Also put to the test will be your application form design, and the validity of your judgements about what's put on it, or on the CV.

INFORMATION FROM THE APPLICATION FORM

If you are wise, you will have made sure that the reply to the form clearly reveals the candidates' possession of the wanted concrete requirements. Some of your criteria will not be concrete, though.

Indicators that could be used to screen application forms for a graduate entry scheme include: intelligence – from examination record; creativity – from 'signs of initiative in work' or 'creative hobbies'; leadership – from 'posts of responsibility at school', rather than 'solitary pursuits'; communication skills – from 'fluent writing, logical and well-argued answers, neat and carefully prepared form'.

Infer from application forms only what is reasonable – do not speculate. Avoid over-interpreting what is said, or marking someone down for what is not there. An interest in amateur theatre may be seen as 'creativity', but in fact it may be an interest in sewing or wiring lights. The person who puts 'reading' may not admit to reading trashy novels. All this begs the question of whether any of this has anything to do with work performance.

There is some unsurprising research evidence that people who write a lot and write neatly are favoured. Many selectors seem to have a preoccupation with the presentation of the form, while others are concerned with matters like family background, which are also of uncertain occupational relevance.

Beware of seeing only what you want to see – of 'interpreting' information on the form in a way that confirms some stereotype, and therefore only reveals your own prejudices.

Here are some of my own predilections. The reader may decide if I show prejudice. I look for evidence of achievement outside work from the work record. I see whether there is evidence here of organising others, and of working in a team, of taking responsibilities, of setting up systems. I look for evidence of unusual aptitudes and things that have required sustained effort. Apart from written communication on the form and what is specifically mentioned by the candidate, I see no point in trying to assess personal skills and personality from what is on the form, with the possible exception of persistence, to which there are sometimes clues.

I do not infer attitudes and values from an application form unless specific questions about these have been asked. As was said in Chapter 17, there is no harm in asking people to make comments about issues in nursing, or about their own strengths and weaknesses, for instance. These can be rated. I ask people to do this briefly – truly a better test of their communication skills than writing an essay. Another common question is to ask them how they meet the requirements of the post.

You can also use the application form to look for patterns to spot gaps and inconsistencies, which may be probed further in

171

the interview, although sometimes they give a strong enough impression to rule someone out. The commonest finding is 'too many different jobs in too short a time'.

USING CRITERIA AS A FRAMEWORK

You should use a grid of criteria to record your shortlisting decisions. Your concern will be to ensure that people are judged as either above or below the line, according to the essential criteria you have derived from the person specification. Needless to say, there should be prior agreement on the criteria and the kind of evidence used. It is no good if a person's many-faceted work record is seen as 'rich and varied' by one person and 'inconsistent' by another.

A shortlisting meeting should be convened, to agree the selection criteria on the basis of the person specification. People can then go away and record evidence for the ratings they give. This exercise will ensure that the panel is clear about what it is looking for, and also standardises its assessment criteria. The panel should be asked to reply quickly, and if there are many candidates and several assessors, you might shortlist those with more than one 'vote'. Alternatively, you could call a second meeting to hammer out differences of view.

The choice of the selection panel should be based on practical requirements. If there are a large number of people who want to participate in selection, you should find some way for them to do this, without being on the shortlisting and interview panel. Give priority for panel membership to people with a direct managerial or professional interest in the post. Medical consultants are often invited to participate in senior clinical appointments, and this is often diplomatically useful, even when they are not quite sure what they are going to ask.

You will also need someone who has professional or technical expertise in the areas where the candidate needs to be assessed. This may be an external assessor, still mandatory for some senior posts. You may find it reassuring to have at least one good probing interviewer present.

REFERENCES

This is often a task that is carried out by the personnel department. Why is it that references are so often not worth the paper they are written on? Often, the process is carried out badly. A standard form is sent to an employer asking for very general information about the candidate's suitability for the post. Relatively few people respond with comprehensive and truthful replies. Everyone is made to appear satisfactory; bad points are omitted or glossed over.

The motivation of managers is sometimes suspect. Consider the well-known scenario of the manager with the unsatisfactory employee she wishes to rid herself of. Providing a bad reference will not achieve this, so a reasonable or non-committal one is offered instead. Furthermore, it is not unknown for a less-than-satisfactory reference to be offered because the manager wants to keep an employee.

Nor are the right people always approached. Friends are not good referees, neither in fact are college tutors who do not know or remember the person's work performance, and who provide a 'reference factory' approach to all enquirers.

It is easy to conceal the truth on paper. Ambiguous statements abound in references. However, people are less guarded on the telephone. You can also probe to ascertain, for example, what people might mean by 'satisfactory'. You can ask frankly whether they would re-employ that person.

How can the reference process be improved? Quite simply, you ask the right questions of the right people at the right time – and in the right way.

The right questions

On paper, you need to ascertain as many as possible of the requirements that you have identified for the job, and to frame them in the form of specific questions. These questions will vary according to the post being applied for, and the current post, but in general you can ask the current manager for her estimation of the person's current performance and of her suitability. The manager may be unwilling to give too many details of the former, and may not be capable of giving you a reliable estimate of the latter.

The following example gives an idea of possible questions for referees. Those marked '*' should be asked in a telephone conversation, rather than on a reference request form.

Example

1 Current post:
- Can you confirm the employment details, including joining date, grade and salary?
- How long has the person been with you?
- Is the person's performance satisfactory?*
- Is the person a committed and reliable employee?*
- What are the person's strengths and weaknesses?*
- Does the person have any special/managerial responsibilities?
- Have there been any problems in the past?*
- What does the person enjoy doing most, and least?*
- Has the person had any difficulty in relating to managers and colleagues, or to patients, clients and relatives?*
- How many days absence has the person had in the past year?
- Has the person been promoted?
- Has the person required correction of any kind?*
- What training has the person received?
- Would the person be considered for promotion?*
- Is there anything else you think we should know about?*
- And the crunch question: Would you re-employ the person in the same job?

2 Post applied for:
- Does the person have skills and knowledge that are likely to be of use?
- Would it appear to be a logical move?
- Is the person capable and ready to take on increased responsibility?
- Do you know of any reason why we should not employ her?*

Some organisations provide a structured questionnaire with yes/no answers. If you adopt this approach, it will be useful to provide space for further comments if necessary.

There is no guarantee that the referee will take the effort you might like, be open with you, or even be a good judge, especially of the candidate's ability to do the new job.

Those who write references regularly are past masters of ambiguity and vagueness, using words like 'average' and 'satisfactory', and stressing areas of strength while omitting the faults, like 'She was a very popular employee' (she did not work because she was always socialising); 'She was most conscientious' (but excruciatingly slow); or 'She had many ideas' (and thought that she could run the place better than the managers).

In order not to allow the person to compose a masterpiece of bland neutrality, it is much better to probe the referee. If she is the person's immediate manager, you can telephone, using the questioning techniques described in Chapter 21 to dig deeper, where appropriate, including asking what, when, where, how and why. If you have probing skills (see Chapter 21), you will want to use them in getting information from referees.

The right people

This means people who know the individual's work well, and preferably manage her.

There may be some good reason why the most obvious person is not listed as a referee. Commonly, it is because the manager has just arrived in post herself. If the direct line manager is not quoted, ask why.

I have never come across any employer getting candidates to ask a subordinate to give a reference, yet someone who has been managed by the individual may have some illuminating remarks on the candidate's management style.

The right time

It is usual in the NHS for references to be taken up when the shortlisting process has been completed. However, there are good arguments for pursuing references only when someone is being offered a position. This saves everyone's time and effort, and the candidate's possible embarrassment later if she fails. If, however, the job has already been offered 'subject to references', it really puts the referee on the line if she does not want to support the candidate. Hence, offering a post 'subject to references' is not to be encouraged.

The other reason for taking up references on shortlisting is so that clues from the references can be used to pursue a particular line of questioning. However, this has its dangers in clumsy hands. At the interview, a lot of stress is put on timekeeping. As a result, it can become obvious that the referee has said something, and in effect the confidentiality is broken. This leads us to the final issue, the etiquette of reference taking.

The right way

It is unethical to approach referees without the candidate's permission. Good employers give applicants the option of whether to allow the referee to be contacted straight away (rare in practice), when shortlisted or only when an offer of a job is made. Remember that in private industry the practice is to ask for a reference only when a job offer has been made.

References are confidential and not to be undertaken lightly. Some managers will be reluctant to complete references, however much they are reassured about confidentiality. The industrial tribunal case of Lawton versus BOC Transhield Limited in 1987 demonstrated that referees may be held liable for negligence, and that their duty of care extends to both the candidate and the recipient.

Confidentiality also means that a reference should not be photocopied to all and sundry. It is recommended practice that one individual maintains the reference, usually the personnel manager. Since the recruiting manager has a 'need to know', she may justify sight of the reference.

The following checklist summarises the steps involved in preliminary screening.

Checklist 20.1

1　Use shortlisting to provide valuable second opinions.
2　Design your paperwork to aid shortlisting.
3　Infer from application forms only what is reasonable – do not speculate.
4　Look for patterns.
5　Use your criteria as a framework.
6　Ensure everyone uses the same criteria.
7　Give priority on the shortlisting panel to those most involved or best equipped to judge.
8　Design reference request forms that will work for you.
9　Ensure the right person is asked the right questions at the right time in the right way.
10　Use the telephone, rather than letters, so that you are able to probe more deeply and get less rehearsed comments.
11　Observe confidentiality and etiquette.

FURTHER READING

Cowan, N and Cowan, R, 'Are references worth the paper they're written on?', *Personnel Management*, December 1989.

Chapter 21

KEY SKILLS FOR THE INTERVIEWER

She had the ability to concentrate totally on what you were saying, as if nothing else in the world mattered. All else vanished, all that existed was you, and what you were telling her.

Kenneth Jupp on Greta Garbo, *The Independent on Sunday*

A great deal has already been said about identifying requirements and person specifications in the previous chapters. The criteria that have been defined are the headings for your summary of evidence form, on which every candidate is to be judged (see Appendix 1). They are also concealed in every question you ask.

GATHERING EVIDENCE USING QUESTIONS

Questions are your tools. The art of questioning goes beyond information gathering. A good question should not only deliver evidence, but lay the ground for obtaining further evidence. Alternatively, it can be used to improve rapport or control. If it does none of these, it is a bad question. So, to develop any level of competence in interviewing, you need to familiarise yourself with the main types of question and know how to use them.

Types of questions

The *open* question does not restrict the answer:

How did you find it?

How do you feel about aggression?

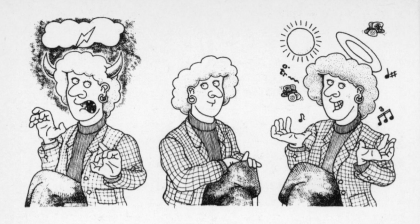

It is designed to give the candidate the opportunity to talk. It usually begins with why, how, what or tell me. Beware of making such a question too open; for example, 'Tell me about yourself. . .' can be disastrous with an over-talkative candidate.

The *closed* question suggests a restricted answer:

Did you find it difficult?

Did you ever have an aggressive patient?

It is used to confirm or sum up a point. It is heavy going to conduct an interview using only closed questions. Some candidates will expand anyway.

The *leading* question signals the answer the interviewer is expecting:

I don't suppose that was too difficult?

I presume that the odd bit of aggression would not worry you, would it?

It provides little evidence, but may be useful occasionally to improve rapport with the candidate. Generally, however, it should be avoided.

The *rhetorical* question is a statement in question form that is not meant to be disputed:

It is deplorable that the nurse should have to face aggression, is it not?

Such a question is often used by people who like to show off to candidates.

The *comparison* question asks the candidate to choose between alternatives:

Do you prefer caring for high or low dependency patients?

It can be useful if the range of comparisons is appropriate.

The *hypothetical* question poses a problem situation for the candidate to respond to:

Would you find that just as difficult here?

How would you cope with an aggressive patient?

The problem is that the candidate is not likely to be aware of local conditions and priorities, so she may dry up, totally baffled. Alternatively, she might, quite innocently, 'get the wrong end of the stick', or give an ideal answer that would not be feasible in practice. A hypothetical question may be used to test textbook knowledge, or imagination. In this case, it may be called a *test* question:

What must a nurse bear in mind when dealing with an aggressive patient?

You must be clear what answer will be acceptable to you when you ask this kind of question – and it should not be so idiosyncratic that even your fellow panel members would not get it right. So the question:

What three things should a nurse always remember?

might have an obvious answer for you, but would completely stump anyone else.

Avoid *multiple* questions, which are really several in one:

Do you have the skills to be able to cope with that kind of thing, and would you enjoy it, or perhaps you would like to develop such skills?

A poor interviewer, often pushed for time, may ask this kind of question. It often stops the candidate in her tracks and damages the rapport. Rarely do you get answers to all the parts.

Probing

A non-probing style is one where there is no attempt to follow up initial questions to dig deeper into the evidence; the candidate's initial response is not followed up. One question is asked on each subject, then the interviewer moves on to the next: 'Do you get on well with people? Have you had to counsel relatives? Have you had to instruct learners? Was this a success?'

The probing interviewer, however, will explore all aspects; for example, whether a 'success' was really what was claimed, whether a claim of achievement by the candidate might have been due to someone else. Probing helps to establish the facts, instead of leaving you with the impressions that the candidate wants you to have.

Probing questions dig deeper. They stretch the candidate. They generate a fuller picture. They ask what?, how? and why? The candidate is invited to reveal what is important, to make useful comparisons, to share her own evaluations: 'Tell me about a time when you had a difficult counselling task? Why was it difficult? What were you aiming to do? Do you feel you succeeded? Why (not)? Would you handle it in the same way again? What kinds of people do you get on best with? Do you prefer to deal with men or women? Why men? What would you say were your strengths with people? Why? Have you developed your ability to influence people during your career? How? Is there anything else? You say "*We* were successful" – what part did *you* play? Was there anything that did not work too well?' Research has suggested that the best guide to future performance is sound evidence about recent past performance. This method is likely to bring you sound evidence, and reveals truths that otherwise might remain hidden.

Questions must not be thought of as isolated items. Think in terms of lines of probing – homing in on the evidence. Start with an open question, then follow with supplementaries, asking why? and how?, to get important details. The following example illustrates this.

Example

Interviewer:	So you found a job in Australia?
Candidate:	Yes, I did.
Interviewer:	What did that involve?
Candidate:	Quite a lot of homework – you know, writing letters, ringing people up, finding people who had been there.
Interviewer:	How many letters did you have to write?
Candidate:	Probably about seventy altogether.
Interviewer:	Why were you so persistent?
Candidate:	I really wanted to go there. In any case, once I put my mind to something, I don't like to give up.
Interviewer:	Was that the only reason?
Candidate:	Well, I was keen on this guy out there and I wanted to join him.

Maybe your reaction is 'This sounds very impressive, but what about when a candidate is not being truthful?'. You may be able to check independently. In the United States, record checking is used considerably, and candidates' awareness of this often forces honesty. If you probe deeply enough, the lack of detail, or of being just 'too good to be true', may make you suspicious. Few people lie outright, but most will tend to play up their achievements. You don't find out if you don't ask.

Probing in depth must be reserved for those occasions where you feel you are likely to get important evidence – not for irrelevancies. You will only be able to probe a maximum of half a dozen things in this way in a half-hour interview. Better, though, to get hard evidence in a few critical areas than superficial evidence in many. Remember also that people learn from experience; what they did in 1971 may not reflect their current approach.

Discovering highlights

It is very useful to ask for the *most* or *least* memorable (or successful, satisfying, interesting, etc.) aspect of a particular experience. This often focuses straight away on something important to the candidate; for example, 'What was the most striking experience you had while nursing in Australia?'.

The following example illustrates further the different kinds of interview question, with comments.

Example

1 Has your health always been good?
   This is not a good question – it is leading and encourages the candidate simply to say 'Yes, it has.' Of course, any detailed probing on health is inappropriate in a selection interview. A better question might be 'How many days sickness have you had in the past year?'.

2 What difficulties would you have in adapting to a computerised system?
   This is rather hypothetical as the person presumably has not had the experience to give other than a speculative answer. If you are assessing this quality of being a good speculator, the question is acceptable. Otherwise, it is better to ask 'What experience have you had with computers?' or 'What difficulties have you found?'.

---

3   Would you rather work on your own?
    The context should be defined. It is a closed question, which
    may be useful if clear alternatives have already been
    discussed and you are now confirming preferences. As a
    starter, however, an open question, like 'How do you feel
    about having to work on your own?', might be better.

4   Would you say you had been successful in your career to
    date?
    This is a leading question that is unlikely to produce an
    uncomplimentary response. It would be better to ask about
    achievements and then, sensitively, about things that did not
    work out or 'development needs'.

5   If you were in Boyle Ward at 5.30 p.m. on a Friday with
    someone waiting to be admitted, a drug round to do and
    several IVs to be put up, what would you do first?
    This is a hypothetical question that is useless if the candidate
    does not have the knowledge to give any kind of answer.

6   In what circumstances might you need to postpone a drug
    round?
    This is better, and is a fair 'test' question.

7   What do you think you would gain professionally from
    moving here?
    This is an open question, containing the assumption that the
    person is interested in her professional development. If this is
    reasonable, then the question is, although it is likely to get a
    rather rehearsed answer.

8   Have you ever had to deal firmly with a visitor?
    Although a closed question, it invites a detailed answer.

9   What happened then?
    This is a follow-up question, used in probing.

See what you think of the following. Try to identify the question
type and whether it is a useful question. Can you improve the
wording? Some suggested improvements are given at the
end.

10 Was this all your own work?

11 What was the worst crisis you have had to deal with in your
    work?

12 Did you get on with your boss?

13 Do you think that your family commitments are likely to
    prevent you attending work at all, or if you moved here and

found that you were unable to have the same kind of help from others, might it be a problem then?

14 You would say you were a self-assured person, would you?

15 What kind of reaction would you expect as a woman supervising men?

16 Are you aware of the opportunities the White Paper presents for us?

17 What are your strengths and weaknesses?

Here are the answers, together with some suggested improvements.

10 A closed question that is a little too leading. It might be better to ask 'What help, if any, did other people give you?'.

11 An open question, of the 'most/least' variety. It is acceptable, if you know that the person will have had to deal with some crises. It may take some time for the candidate to locate it in her mind – some candidates may say 'I can't really think of one.'

12 A closed, leading question, to which the answer will be 'yes', making it hard to probe without appearing suspicious of the answer. It might be better to say 'We all have differences of opinion with our bosses at times. When was the last time you disagreed with yours?' Then probe.

13 A horrendous multiple question that needs to be broken up. The first question could be rephrased as 'What support do you find you need in order to work and meet your family commitments?'. Then, perhaps, 'Do you know whether you would be able to get that support here?'. This is clearly a dangerous area to be questioning (see Chapter 19).

14 A closed, leading question, used to confront the candidate. Said more for effect than to get evidence.

15 A hypothetical question, with discriminatory overtones.

16 Closed in form, and leading, because the questioner obviously wants an answer that agrees with her view. It might be better to ask 'Do you think the White Paper offers opportunities?' and then probe 'What are they?' and 'Why?'.

17 Multiple, open question. Best to ask about each separately.

The following checklist gives hints on using questions.

LISTENING

Some have said that this is the most important skill of all. Look as if you are listening; listen for content, but listen for deeper meanings as well. It is not easy. Without notes, you will forget and distort what is said. Aim to let the candidate talk relevantly for 80% or 90% of the time.

It is harder to listen properly if you are remembering your own script, if you are not asking the questions for a long time, or if the candidate's style is boring.

RAPPORT

You will want to develop trust and facilitate disclosure in a relaxed atmosphere. Here are some things that make for good rapport.

Active listening involves showing the candidate that you are doing so by maintaining eye contact (at least for 25% of the time – you may not need more); by encouraging and sensitively summarising and echoing what is said, when appropriate. Use pauses constructively, not awkwardly. This is the essence of maintaining rapport. However, its level depends on many other things, and can be broken instantly.

What do your interview arrangements say to the candidate? The seating arrangements may speak of your superiority. The likelihood of interruption, or the rushed pace, may be a signal that she is not really important. Uncomfortable surroundings may unnerve the candidate. Formality may be off-putting. Give the candidate space, in every sense.

Personal touches, like having one of the panel collect the candidate, acknowledging her anxieties, addressing her frequently by first name, will help. The start of the interview can be

184

made gentle, friendly and relaxing, or stiff and inhibiting. Too much joviality and familiarity may seem phoney, however.

State the purpose and the timings of the interview. Will it be a hundred yard sprint or a marathon?

The odd embarrassing or too personal remark, when assumptions and prejudices are given too much rein, can be damaging. The atmosphere can suddenly freeze, and the candidate may become defensive, or the conversation may dry up. The interviewers should match the level of vocabulary of the candidate. They should give approval where possible, especially for openness and revelations by the candidate, and should never show shock or disapproval. However, I have noticed that good interviewers are not afraid to project pleasure or disappointment at times.

British interviewers tend to be too nice, at times artifically nice, hiding their own nervousness and their fears of confronting the candidate. The result is rather insipid interviewing. Often, a confident candidate can manipulate this situation, and ensure that no negative note is ever introduced.

So, do allow a little of your personality and feeling to show. However, there is nothing worse, I am sure you will agree, than an interviewer (usually male) on an ego trip, who is showing off to the panel and candidate. You can confront without antagonising – 'Perhaps I might ask. . .?' and 'Could there be. . .' are useful leads.

Explain that you will be taking notes. Do it fairly openly, but make sure that you give the candidate your full attention when she is saying something important. Do not rush to take notes immediately something striking is said. Wait a minute or two. Note the content, not your opinion.

The following checklist gives hints on listening and achieving rapport.

Checklist 21.2

1 Listen actively – show you are listening.
2 Aim to let the candidate talk for 80% of the time.
3 Active listening helps rapport.
4 The environment tells the candidate a lot.
5 Match the candidate's openness.
6 Be yourself, a little – do not be too formal or too informal.
7 Put the candidate in the picture about what is happening.
8 Take notes openly.

CONTROL

You are no dictator. However, you need to ensure certain outcomes, and you will want the means to bring the interview to heel at times. This may mean controlling your own performance or the candidate's.

Interviewing often feels like balancing a number of spinning plates. It involves a simultaneous demonstration of all of the competencies described here, all the time monitoring and adjusting what you are doing. Inexperienced interviewers dry up. They forget what they should be doing and hand over to a colleague, blushingly revealing their incompetence. If this is your problem, do not worry. You will learn to hide this by saying weakly 'Thank you, that's all for the time being, but I'd like the chance to come back later.'

Some inexperienced interviewers stumble in their panic into awful leading questions, like 'That wouldn't be a problem for you, would it?', 'Do you think you could cope with. . .' or 'Your health is no problem, is it?', forgetting to add the instruction to quantify, by asking 'To what extent. . .' or 'What problems would you see. . .'. Others ask terrifying multiple questions, which reduce the candidate to silence instead. With wisdom, you will learn the pitfalls, and learn to pause and break up the questions into manageable portions. Control does come with experience, and even good interviewers lose tight control of their performance occasionally.

If you know where you are in the interview (because you have prepared, and/or developed the skills with practice), you can achieve control by using very simple devices. You can gently stop the candidate and slow the pace by reflecting back on what she has said. You can refer back to something said previously, or use linking questions, like 'You mentioned driving just now, do you drive yourself?'.

How do you control the candidate, when you need to? Is the person too dominant or too talkative, or is she referring to irrelevant issues? Roughly, in order of severity, you might try any of the following. Using body language (lean forward or even withdraw), disengage eye contact and say 'Yes, yes, yes. . .' while nodding furiously. Say 'very briefly' when you invite the candidate to talk. Glance at your watch, say 'Yes, that's very interesting. . .' (about the travels in Khandahar, or views on the future of the NHS) '. . .but I'd like to get back to talking about the wards you have managed.' Use closed, rather than open questions. Say you are not happy with the way she is responding and that it is not helping the purpose of the interview, and that unfortunately time is limited and the next candidate is waiting . . . frown . . . .

For the shy candidate, you will need to be patient, improve the rapport, ask open questions, use an encouraging tone of voice, and allow time to respond. It is always helpful to ask *why* the candidate is behaving as she is. This will reveal your tactics – but you will need to have a repertoire of verbal and non-verbal responses available.

You will not want to be interrupted by other panel members. A steely glare can do the trick for you, but the candidate may notice. If there is a panel, it must be properly co-ordinated and the ground rules established beforehand.

The person chairing a panel will be expected to control the proceedings and to stop the interviewer who goes on too long, usually by subtle means, but not always. The 'free for all' approach irritates those who construct careful lines of questions like chess openings, and they do not want others jumping in and wrecking it. But some panels help each other out well. Remember that unexpected interventions may throw the candidate; you will often find the person having to glance around the room as if she were under the umpire's chair at Wimbledon.

Perhaps the hardest thing to control is timing. I have never yet known a series of interviews to run on time. Parkinson's Law operates. While some panels are inefficient, I have sympathy with the panel that overruns by a few minutes to get that vital piece of evidence.

The skills outlined in this chapter are all interdependent. A poor misunderstood question, or faulty listening, will affect the rapport. You may then lose control and fail to get the evidence you need. The following checklist highlights how to keep control.

Checklist 21.3

1 Achieve control through good preparation.
2 Use verbal and non-verbal signals.
3 Avoid 'free for alls' – observe the ground rules.
4 Remember timing.

PREPARATION

This will include all the interview arrangements, before, during and after. All parties must be in no doubt as to how things are to happen, and they must have full details in writing of times, venue, jobs, candidates and person specifications. The criteria should come as no surprise to anyone. Questions of salary, terms and conditions, promotion prospects and non-pay benefits must be covered, and everyone must know to whom to refer them.

The panel should have a generous timetable, with space for lunch, tea and coffee breaks. Scheduling more than six interviews in a day is not advised, as fatigue effects are bound to blur judgements. Needless to say, the room must be quiet and free from interruptions.

I like to give the candidates as much information in a letter of invitation as I can. This will include details of the panel, and other candidates. Candidates should be given a comfortable room to wait in, with coffee offered at the beginning. You might well want to invite them to look around, or to read. If things get delayed, tell them, explaining why. There is no harm in their meeting members of the panel before the interview, or having lunch with them. However, it is usually as well to allow them to go home straight after the interview, if you can.

You will need to communicate the arrangements for notifying the decision, and whether any feedback will be available to candidates.

You will want to ensure that all of your resources are in place, and that everyone, from the switchboard to the general manager, is aware of your schedule, including last minute changes.

An interview report form will help structure peoples' judgements and provide you with some documentation of the basis for the decisions. Since commitment and discipline are required to complete such forms, and such habits are not often well established, it is as well to keep them simple. I favour a simple form that asks for evidence, and assessment ratings, against each criterion. One form is completed by each interviewer for each candidate.

The interviewers will have some idea of the questions they are going to ask – at least as starting points. Structured interviews are better than unstructured ones, but over-structured interviews can be too rigid. Why not send out a questionnaire instead? You will need to be flexible and explore the unexpected leads.

Some people think that lists of criteria can be used to provide a structure for the interview; for example, 'I'll ask about motivation, you ask about relationships, then he'll ask about leadership.' This is crude and unmanageable. Evidence on each criteria will often emerge in several areas. The interview structure should be based on subject areas that make sense to the candidate, as well as the panel.

Panels are not inevitable. They do give a shared experience and time out for silent observation. Sequential, one-to-one interviews covering different aspects (using the same criteria) are just as reliable, a lot quicker, and preferred by candidates. The rapport is usually better. You may want to use one interview as a screening interview – you should avoid decisions being made by a sole individual, however, as this could be discriminatory.

Finally, give some thought to the interview arrangements. Interviewing across a desk is not welcoming, neither is having four or five people squashed into a room eight feet square. Try out the seating arrangements by taking the candidate's position. Ensure that it feels comfortable, that the candidate has some freedom of movement, and that it is neither too close nor too remote from the interviewers. Chapter 11 gives some hints on what to avoid.

The following checklist summarises the steps involved in preparation.

Checklist 21.4

1 Is the schedule clear and has adequate time been given?
2 Is there some leeway for possible delays?
3 Have all of those involved been briefed?
4 Have all interruptions been precluded?
5 Is all of the documentation ready, including schedules, application forms, references, job descriptions, person specifications, interview report forms, salary details, references, travel claim forms, etc?
6 Has the panel prepared its approach together – consensus on requirements and criteria, who will be doing what?

FURTHER READING

Anderson, N and Shackleton, V, 'Recruitment and selection: a review of developments in the 1980s', *Personnel Review*, **15**(4), 1986.

Goodale, James G, *The Fine Art of Interviewing* (Prentice-Hall, 1982).

Goodworth, Clive T, *Effective Interviewing for Employment Selection* (Business Books, 1979).

Grummit, Janis, *A Guide to Interviewing Skills* (Industrial Society, 1980).

Higham, M, *The ABC of Interviewing* (IPM, 1979).

IDS, *Race and Sex Discrimination: Interviewing and Selection* (IDS, Brief No. 325, 1986).

Lock, Harold F, *Interviewing for Selection*, 4th Edn (National Institute for Industrial Psychology, 1972).

MacKay, Ian, *A Guide to Asking Questions* (British Association for Commercial and Industrial Education, 1980).

Mackenzie, Davey, D and McDonnell, P, *How to Interview* (British Institute of Management, 1975).

Rae, L, *The Skills of Interviewing* (Gower, 1988).

Roberts, Celia, *The Interview Game and How It's Played* (BBC, 1985).

Chapter 22

GATHERING EVIDENCE – ASSESSMENT AGAINST CRITERIA

Judge not by the appearance.   *Gospel according to St John*

It is only shallow people who do not judge by appearances.
                                                         Oscar Wilde

Never allow yourself to be swept off your feet: when an impulse stirs, see first that it will meet the claims of justice; when an impression forms, assure yourself first of its certainty.
                                         Marcus Aurelius, *Meditations*

This chapter brings together the person specification and the selection methods in order to create an interview plan. We will look at sources of evidence in general, and also at how the questioning techniques studied in the last chapter can be used to obtain evidence in areas where criteria have been specified. We will use the CCR scheme, as explained in Chapter 16.

COMPETENCE

Sources of evidence

The application form or CV will of course provide evidence of qualifications and experience. This will often be written to give a good impression, and will omit any weaknesses. The experience may suggest that the person has acquired certain skills, but you cannot make assumptions. Hence, you will need to probe further at the interview for evidence of concrete achievement and for gaps. A structured application form or reference will help you home in on what you are looking for (see Chapter 20).

Sample interview approach

Direct questions:

- What were your responsibilities?
- What training did you have?
- What did you learn from that?
- Would you do the same thing again?
- How did you tackle that?
- What are your strengths?
- What are your development needs?
- Could you teach other people in that area?

Test question:

- What do you think important in. . .? (state the situation)

Probing approaches:

- What did you find (technically) most difficult? Why was that? What was the problem? Have you developed an approach to such problems since then? Have you tried it out? How effective was your approach?
- We have all been in situations where things did not go according to plan. Can you describe a situation where you faced this problem? (then probe as above)
- Can you give me an example of a situation that brought out all of your skills as a nurse? What happened? (etc.)
- You say that you have done ward budgets. What did that involve? (etc.)

COMMITMENT CRITERIA

Interests

Sources of evidence

The application form or CV will provide clues. Then, in the interview, you can assess the depth.

Sample interview approach

Direct questions:

- What aspects of. . . interest you? Why is that? How have you pursued those interests?
- What have you read?

- What courses have you attended?
- Why did you choose those options?

In most cases, the answers will be factual and easily volunteered. If the candidate is bluffing to impress, keep probing, testing her knowledge and experience, and ask her opinions about issues:

- Give me your views on... (topical issues).
- Do you agree with...? Why do you say that?

Compatibility

Sources of evidence

The enthusiasm or otherwise of the referee may provide a clue. You can see from the application form or CV whether the person has tended to stay within organisations, or has been promoted. However, there is little that will be reliable evidence here. In fact, you should be very wary.

You may get favourable impressions if the person gives you signals than indicate 'our kind of person'. This could be a 'gut feeling' that you warm to her – often because she smiles and talks enthusiastically – or because she hits the right note on the application, or even because she has had the same training as one of the interviewers. Beware of this 'halo effect' (see Chapter 11). Do not get carried away by superficial information. There may be some hidden areas of incompatibility, or you may be being manipulated by a clever candidate.

In the interview, you must establish the candidate's preferences from the choices she has made in her life and career. This is an area in which the candidate has a real interest in co-operating with you. However, this will often conflict with a desire to impress, and wanting to give you the message 'I am the person you want'.

Sample interview approach

Establish good rapport and try to get the candidate talking frankly about her preferences.

Direct questions:

- Why did you leave?
- Why did you take this (next) job?

- What is important to you (in your job)?
- Why do you want to work here?
- What kind of management style do you have?
- What kinds of people do you prefer to work with?
- What kinds of people do you find it difficult to work with?
- What were the differences between this job and the other one?

Probing approaches:

- Why do you say that?
- Is that the only thing?
- Are you sure that is what you want?
- Do you think you will find that (what you want) here?

Confidence

Sources of evidence

Obtain as much information as you can from the referees. A very positive reference will be reassuring; a hesitant one, worrying.

Does the application form suggest sudden changes of direction? Reasons for leaving jobs that are mentioned on the application form may give you some clues. This must be probed. In the interview, you need to check the candidate's reliability when given responsibility.

Sample interview approach

Some of the candidate's preferences (see earlier) may provide a clue; for example, 'What kind of supervision do you like to have?'.

Talk about relationships – you need to be subtle. 'Would you be able to cope?' is poor, and leading.

Direct questions:

- What kinds of people do you get on best with?
- If you were ever to have a disagreement with a colleague (a doctor?), what would it likely to be about?

Probing approach:

- Have you ever been asked to do something that you felt to be unreasonable. . . (or against your principles)?

Pick up (gently and sympathetically) any suggestion of difficulty with superiors or colleagues, or failure to achieve. 'That must have been difficult?' Encourage the candidate to give you her analysis. 'Why do you think your colleague seemed so obstructive?' If you get too much self-justification, or she runs down her last boss, you may suspect a lack of self-awareness. You might follow with 'How did you cope with that?'. The answer may suggest rigidity – or too much accommodation of others.

Application

Sources of evidence

A pattern of achievement is often apparent in many candidates' CVs. You may also spot gaps and rather arbitrary decisions they have made. You need to know what a candidate has achieved overall, and find some examples of particular successes.

Sample interview approach

Direct questions:

- What did you achieve in that job?
- What objectives were you set?
- To what extent did you achieve them?
- What help did you get?
- What made you give up eventually?

Probe successes critically and failures sympathetically, so that you can start to identify the person's own contribution from that of the prevailing winds of fortune, or the icy hand of fate. Identify where support was strong, and where it was lacking.

Circumstances

Sources of evidence

Generally, you are constrained to what the candidate is prepared to disclose. If circumstances impinge on health, then you must leave the assessment to your occupational health department.

Opportunities for exploring circumstances will often arise when issues are raised by the candidate – for example, about accommodation – outside of the interview. It may be the role of the personnel officer to check this out. Disclosure of criminal convictions will be sought on the application form.

Sample interview approach

There is a limited scope for questioning. I believe it is reasonable to ask all candidates:

- Are there circumstances in your private life that might make it difficult for you to attend with perfect regularity/work late sometimes?

Here, the relevance to the job is obvious, without suspicion of sex bias or assumptions about children.

CLASSIFYING EVIDENCE AGAINST CRITERIA

Do not use the criteria list as a list of interview topic headings. If you do, your intentions will be spotted a mile off by the candidate, even if you don't actually say 'Let's look at your commitment to this job' or 'Let's explore your personality'.

A criteria-based interview assessment form is given in Appendix 1. I recommend that you use something like this, but do not try to classify the evidence while you are interviewing. Take rough notes on what the candidate says and classify later. We will look at the use of notes in Chapter 24.

Table 22.1 is a summary chart, showing how evidence can be classified against criteria.

Table 2?.1 Using selection methods in gathering evidence against criteria

Criteria	Selection Method			
	Application form/CV	References	Interview	Tests
Competence	Possibly through jobs done and promotions	Of immediate supervisors – may be easier to collect positive rather than negative evidence	Use structured probing to get behind what is said to impress	Only appropriate if a suitable validated test is used
Commitment Interests	Possibly	Unlikely	Good because not threatening – probe to test depth	Only useful for vocational guidance
Compatibility Confidence	May be clues in job changes	Unlikely on paper – more likely when probed on the telephone	Clues can be followed up through subtle probing	May be detectable through a personality inventory
Application	Study track record – more likely to include successes rather than failures	Best to probe referee on the telephone	Need to probe closely to check that stated achievement really happened and was not due to others' efforts	Learning can be tested
Circumstances	There may be clues – it is dangerous to infer too much	Generally, inappropriate to ask	Need to observe equal opportunity principles – may pursue issues mentioned and ask about job-related issues	Not appropriate

Chapter 23

INTERVIEWING INTERNAL CANDIDATES

He hath better bettered expectation than you must expect of me to tell you how. Shakespeare, *Much Ado About Nothing*

AN OBVIOUS MATCH?

Perhaps you believe that you have the ideal replacement for your vacancy already – someone who has strong expectations of taking over. Promises have not been made explicitly, but if your individual performance reviews (IPRs) are working, then that person will know where she stands. This may give you an enormous sense of relief. However, if you have any doubts, and a threat has been made to the effect that 'I'll leave if I don't get that job', you will need to stand firm.

When Len Peach was NHS Chief Executive, he made no secret of his belief in succession planning. However, NHS tradition has always been that of open competition. As a result, people make fruitless trips to the far ends of the country, only to find that they are being used as yardsticks to measure the internal candidate.

Staff may feel resentful if the internal applicant is not appointed, particularly if that person has been 'acting up'.

Consideration of whether the candidate matches the requirements must be done fairly and objectively. Others in the unit or district, who are waiting for an opportunity to show what they can do, must also be included.

No one should underestimate the difficulties of interviewing fairly and effectively, and of ensuring that the right person gets the job. Never is this more true than when internal candidates are involved.

USING WHAT YOU ALREADY KNOW

Let us consider the assessment of an internal candidate, call him George. George is the candidate for the post he is currently acting in, which involves recruitment of staff. He has had to make the interview arrangements for this appointment. His boss is on the panel. George enters the room, introduces himself as the recruitment officer and announces that there is one candidate for this particular post – himself. He then brings in the papers for the panel, including his own references, one of which is from his boss. He then re-enters the room as the candidate. He is interviewed, then leaves, shortly to return with coffee for the panel. He asks them to let him know when they have made their decision. Eventually, they make the decision – not to offer him the post.

This scenario raises several issues. Firstly, internal candidates should be assessed quite separately from their normal work situation. You should consider whether they need to be assessed at all. If IPR is working, it will have indicated George's readiness for promotion, and a succession planning system will have indicated George's possible next move. It may then be a simple job of bringing in an outside assessor, and perhaps a colleague to test the boss's judgement. Psychometric assessment may be appropriate, as it is so objective.

The dilemma where internal candidates are involved is that, on the one hand, you want to put internal candidates over the same set of hurdles as other people, so you are seen to be fair to everyone. Yet, on the other hand, you do know the individual's strengths and weaknesses, so the interview will seem superfluous or artificial. If the internal candidate then fails the hurdles, the feelings of resentment will increase.

You should make use of what you know already about internal candidates. Do not put them through embarrassing ritual hoops when you already have evidence of what you are looking for. You may need to get others to confirm this. You may need to have professional competence checked by an assessor. You may need to know where your candidate stands in relation to others. The candidate should be kept informed of the process, and of possible outcomes, throughout.

We return here to the interviews of Michael Davis and Tony Brown, which were described from the candidate's point of view in Chapter 12. Here, we will look at the situation from the panel's point of view.

Case study

Alberton Hospital has introduced a number of procedures to attempt to make the interview process less hit and miss. Every candidate who now applies is given a detailed person specification describing the criteria for the job. And in this particular case, all candidates were asked to fill out a detailed questionnaire assessing how the interview had gone. They were also offered post-interview counselling.

The fact that all of the candidates for the jobs were internal and that, at the end of the process, the panel agreed that only two people met all of the criteria, would suggest that the interviews were relatively straightforward. But the truth is, no interview is straightforward.

A week later, when I talked to the interview panel, consisting of a personnel officer, a nurse manager, a tutor and a clinical psychologist, it revealed a far from simple route to appointment.

For a start, there was the process of shortlisting. A total of nine people applied for the two jobs, one of whom withdrew at an early stage. The rest were shortlisted, despite the fact that the panel had serious reservations about a couple of the candidates. 'We had agreed that if the applicant was on the borderline, we'd give him the benefit of the doubt,' said personnel officer Jill Johnston, 'but we never got together again to discuss these marginal cases. I think if we had, maybe things would have been different.'

They also learnt a fortuitous lesson about the optimum number to interview. Originally, the panel had intended to interview eight candidates at hourly intervals between 9.00 a.m. and 6.00 p.m. But this was reduced to six because of withdrawals. 'I think six in a day is the maximum,' said clinical psychologist Mary Roberts, 'I was involved in eight interviews a day for three days once, and it was absolutely mind-boggling.'

Agreeing, Jill commented: 'I think you start to flag when there is no break.' The withdrawal of two candidates gave the panel the necessary breathing space.

The mechanics of the interview were carefully arranged to ensure fairness and impartiality. Each member of the panel asked a series of pre-arranged questions, which were then followed up with supplementary, unrehearsed questions to tease out information that did not emerge from the first round.

Again, in retrospect, the panellists felt that some of their questions had not been clear enough. In particular, Wendy Smith, the nurse manager, regretted one question that she had asked all of the candidates: What is the difference between management and leadership? 'Most of the candidates seemed non-plussed by the question, so I don't think I would ask it like that again.'

One well-known pitfall is drawing conclusions about a candidate prematurely and then using the rest of the interview to confirm those prejudices. All panellists were aware of this danger, but believed they had avoided the trap. 'In a couple of cases, I started out more favourably inclined than I finished up', noted Mary.

'One candidate I thought was doing very well,' agreed Jill, 'but the further the interview progressed the more faults I started to find in the person's performance.'

On the face of it, the two candidates focused on represented the two ends of the spectrum. Michael Davis had not had an interview for 10 years, and in the words of one interviewer, 'failed the criteria I had listed on at least five or six counts'.

Tony Brown had been a senior nurse manager at the hospital until two years ago, only to be regraded to charge nurse as the result of an internal re-organisation. The team leader job was equivalent to the management position he had previously held.

It was clear that Michael's curriculum vitae had been so poor that he had been lucky to get past the starting post. Handwritten in pale blue ink, it was rambling, unpunctuated and disorganised. 'It was the sort of application that I would have expected from a more junior person: it omitted anything about management or supervisory aspects.'

'I wasn't sure whether he understood the job properly,' said Jill, 'even though he must have read the job specification.'

'I got the feeling from the curriculum vitae that his work wasn't client centred — it seemed to involve doing things to people rather than enabling people to develop in their own way', commented tutor Alan Wells.

Wendy found the colour of the ink and the fact that she could not read parts of the text particularly irritating, which raises the question — Should interviewers make judgements on the basis of what seem to be incidentals? Wendy Smith was convinced they should: 'I think it is quite justified if the job is a responsible one and the work involves presentation.'

'It's not so much whether it is handwritten or typed but how it is presented,' observed Jill, 'the important thing is that it should be divided into a logical sequence of events and broken up under headings.'

In many ways, the interview bore out the misgivings of some of the panellists about shortlisting Michael in the first place. Although he conducted himself well and revealed a conscientious personality, he showed no awareness of managing people. 'He was very clear about how to help staff,' said Wendy 'but he didn't seem able to identify any process he would use to consciously achieve that.' He had difficulty in identifying any understanding of a problem-solving approach to his work.

'We were looking for some sort of evaluation of the service being provided, but he found it hard to tell us what made it work or not work. I felt that here is someone who has an overwhelming willingness and flexibility, but in the end he would be doing everything, and his staff would be doing nothing', said Jill.

So, was it a mistake to shortlist him in the first place? Alan, one of those who was least impressed by Michael's curriculum vitae, nevertheless felt that the interview had been worthwhile. 'I felt that it was a good experience for him. I was pleased that we brought him in because he has certainly demonstrated a lot of accomplishments over the years, and that really came across strongly. I felt that the potential was there. He was very responsive and alive, very endearing. The difficulty was applying that to the person needed for this particular job.'

'I had the impression that if you set him things to do, he'd probably go ahead and do them,' commented Jill, 'but at the moment he's a follower, not a leader. The question for us now is to see whether we can turn the tables and develop his leadership qualities.'

Wendy Smith, however, did not agree. 'If he's interested in practice, let's help him in that and work on his strong points.'

For Tony Brown, the other candidate, leadership qualities posed no problem, and the panel had no doubts that, on the basis of his curriculum vitae, he should be shortlisted for the job. His application was well organised, clear and polished – the only adverse comment was that the person portrayed in it bore little resemblance to the one who presented himself at the interview.

This is, incidentally, an important issue. There is little point in producing a superb curriculum vitae that you cannot back up at the interview. As Jill Johnston commented: 'You can get very expert writers who just don't perform at the interview.'

The converse is also true. Alan Wells said: 'Many qualities are difficult to detect in written form, yet they come out so clearly in successful candidates and are so obviously absent in unsuccessful ones.'

'The interview itself began promisingly. He started off really brilliantly,' said Wendy, 'talking about how he had gone into this ward, and describing very clearly how he and his team of staff had identified deficits in the service.'

'He displayed very early on an ability to identify what actually mattered. For instance, he talked about the patients' lack of privacy, lack of contact and lack of material possessions, and he described how one of his first acts was to ensure that every patient had his own comb.'

'He displayed a good understanding of what was wrong with the service and described how the staff team negotiated together over what they would prioritise. He immediately identified how you make things happen.'

'You could tell he was in control of things because the answers weren't too lengthy,' noted Jill, 'sometimes his answers were quite short.'

'Although he could not identify staff development, he conveyed that he used his personality to develop enthusiasm among others', said Wendy. 'Obviously, that sort of approach raised some questions, but the panel asked him what happened when that approach didn't work and his reply was simple: "I've never had problems." '

'And,' commented Alan, 'it was said in such a way that we believed him.'

It was at this stage that the mood of the interview changed. Wendy again: 'I felt he had some off-putting mannerisms. He was very low down in his chair and it was almost as though he was a bit arrogant. He made one or two glib and inappropriate jokes, and then he was a bit sharp with Mary. I felt he was getting rather argumentative – then he quietened down again.'

Interestingly, the panel was divided on how to interpret this behaviour. Alan has known Tony Brown for over 10 years and is very sensitive to how the health service has treated people like him during that time. He interpreted Tony's anger during the interview as an anger about his past treatment and, therefore, not something to be worried about.

For Wendy Smith, however, that is not the point. 'I can understand the anger, but I just don't think you should show it at an interview – it's not appropriate. He will need to be very careful about this in future.'

When it came to discussing Tony's credentials for the job, both Wendy and Jill expressed concern about his behaviour during the interview, but they were eventually won over by Alan and Mary. 'I just got the feeling that he recognised that he had a short fuse and wasn't going to let it get in the way', commented Jill.

'When he talked about himself, he talked about persistence and stubbornness,' noted Wendy, 'that somehow made his behaviour in the interview more understandable. I think the truth is that he doesn't like talking about himself – and that's the way he shows it.'

Did the panel consider asking Tony why he was behaving in such a confrontational manner? 'No,' said Jill, 'he was clearly on edge and I think if we had raised it, the situation would have worsened.'

It is interesting, however, that the outside assessor felt that Tony's attitude was the least satisfactory part of the interview. 'My initial impression was here is a very, very angry man who wants to know why he should have had to apply for this job', said Sally Colter of the Raine Partnership consultancy. She noted an entirely different atmosphere in this interview, as compared with the others. 'His manager had been quite relaxed through the other interviews, but she took on a very different stance in this one. The body language of the panel changed completely. Their knees hunched up, the clipboards came out and the arms were folded.'

Things came to a head when, in response to one question from Mary, Tony sharply turned the question back on her. It marked the tensest moment of a difficult interview, and, according to Sally Colter, Mary seemed to lose interest in the interview after this exchange.

Sally also felt that the fact that the panellists knew the candidate meant they were less able to cope with his anger and to assess its significance afterwards. 'I was not surprised that he got the job – my gut feeling was that it was almost a foregone conclusion. But if I were an external examiner, I would have wanted to probe more deeply into what the aggression meant – and whether it would spill over into the ward. I also wondered about his motivation for the job.'

She also claimed that Tony was the only candidate to be quizzed in depth about his past experience. This was rejected by the panel. 'All candidates were asked about their past experience', said Wendy. 'Tony expanded more on his past work, but he was certainly not asked more.'

Nor had they made up their mind about him in advance – as testified by the long discussion after the interview – and their previous knowledge of him had not coloured their views.

At least one panellist made it clear that she was not too worried by Tony's behaviour at the interview, because it had never shown itself in the ward. Could she have made such a generous assessment of an outside candidate who exhibited similar attitudes during an interview? In the light of this, Sally Colter's suggestion that an external examiner should sit in on all internal interviews, at least for nurse managers, seems a sensible one. As she says: 'I can't see how you can help making assumptions about candidates you know.'

As to whether the panel chose the right candidate for the job, time alone will tell. The fact that Tony is in his new post seems to dispel Sally's initial fear that he was not really interested in the job. But it is still early days.

Conversely, the panel clearly made the right decision not to appoint Michael Davis. But were they right to shortlist him in the first place? Has the whole process further dented his confidence?

Ultimately, those may be unanswerable questions, but they demonstrate what a difficult job the interview panel faces and how far-reaching the consequences are of getting it wrong. Who, indeed, would be an interviewer?

The following checklist gives guidance on interviewing internal candidates.

Checklist 23.1

1 Tell internal candidates as much about the process of selection as possible. You may need to make this information available to other candidates as well. If there is an internal re-organisation, make sure that everyone knows the procedures. Make sure that the candidate has every opportunity to prepare well.

2 Where possible, ensure that some appraisal has taken place with the candidate, that lets her know where she stands.

3 Do not encourage people to apply simply 'for the experience'. This can be damaging.

4 Where possible, see internal candidates separately from outsiders. This may involve a separate screening interview. Make sure that they are completely free from their work commitments on that day.

5 Ensure that an external assessor is involved, and that she can be assured that the process is fair. She must be allowed to ask whatever questions she wants to, of and about the internal candidate.

6 Utilise all sound evidence you already have about the candidate, and make this available, maybe in the form of a confidential reference or internal record of competency.

7 Make plans to give internal candidates good feedback on the decision, and support in coming to terms with failure.

Chapter 24

COMING TO A DECISION

His conversation usually threatened and announced more than it performed: that he fed you with a continual renovation of hope to end in a constant succession of disappointment.

Dr Samuel Johnson

WHAT WENT WRONG?

If you have done a lot of interviewing, you will have made some mistakes – perhaps picked a few people who did not live up to their promise, or who were outright disasters. You will, no doubt, have rejected some good people, snapped up later by others.

There was no hint of the personality problems at the interview.

I had my doubts about her at the time, but I was in a minority.

She said she could do it, but it turned out to be all talk.

We were all taken in at the interview, she came across as superb.

I thought we had another Margaret here, but I was so wrong.

I would like to return to our scenario on page 115, where Mrs Garnett and Miss Williams were interviewing Sally. Note their conclusions carefully. Do you think they were justified?

Mrs Garnett obtained factual information about Sally's career to date, but she did not probe deeply. This meant that she knew a lot about what Sally says she did, but not about how well she did it. The questions with obvious answers, like 'Would you

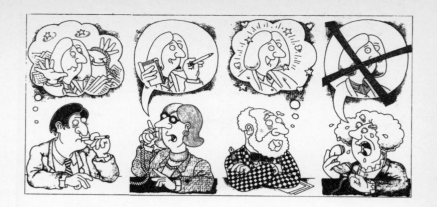

mind taking charge?', 'Are you confident about your clinical knowledge?' and 'Could you cope with the pressures here?', enabled Sally to give the required answer, and produced little evidence of her capability, only of her being streetwise enough to say what was obviously required.

Miss Williams indicated that she had found this young lady wanting. Despite the attempt to gloss over her faults, Miss Williams felt that she had detected them. Everything pointed to the fact that Sally was not of the calibre required, certainly not up to the standard of the person they had seen last week. All the evidence pointed one way.

Miss Williams had set out to collect as much negative information as she could, and very little of a positive nature. She therefore might have a rather distorted picture. Miss Williams also made some false assumptions when Sally was talking about her relationship with the sister she trained with – the evidence here must be suspect, although Miss Williams would not be aware that the data is capable of a different interpretation from the one she gives it. Having set up a false impression, Miss Williams tended to look for any evidence to confirm her views, and ignored anything that contradicted it.

Sally's hesitancy later on was taken to mean that she was clinically incompetent, rather than simply flustered by the intimidation she felt in the unfamiliar interview situation.

Remember what I said earlier about their methods of arriving at their decision. They did not discuss the qualities they wanted, the criteria, or the standards. They did not discuss how they were going to get evidence. They probably had some intuitive or stereotyped ideas of the person they were looking for, but they did not make them objective, and we did not know whether they shared these ideas.

Any criteria they did use were in their heads, and they might find it hard to explain them. They did not discuss the candidates in relation to criteria, but merely compared one person with another, in rather vague subjective terms. Impressions were allowed to rule their judgement.

In the end, their decision was based on a very subjective reaction. It included some untested assumptions about the candidate. They thought they had evidence, but they ended up merely trying to justify their initial subjective impressions.

Mrs Garnett preferred to keep to factual information, but was not sure how to evaluate the information she received. She certainly did not probe the candidate. She really would admit that she had little basis for selection. 'Why do I choose this one rather than that one? I am not really sure. As she has given better answers to my questions, I think she would be rather more organised on the ward.'

Miss Williams, on the other hand, was highly judgemental. She regularly found herself going beyond the factual evidence. She made inferences and relied a lot on 'gut reaction'. This, for her, was her special art – weighing people up. It is what made her a good interviewer in her opinion. 'There was something about that last candidate that I did not care for – perhaps it was her style of dress. She seemed a bit too forward – I am sure she would have given us trouble.'

Neither were aware of their mistakes, and they would probably not have much idea what to do about them, if they did know.

OBTAINING GOOD EVIDENCE

Here are some rules for getting good evidence.

Know what to look for

Much has been said about this already. The main point is to be able to set sound criteria.

Obtain adequate information related to the criteria set

Everything you know officially about a person is usable. What is in the application form and references is potential evidence. In terms of the interview, you need to probe as deeply as you can – to get beneath the superficial impressions that you have, or the candidate wishes you to have. You need to seek information that can be used as evidence. It is dangerous to judge on impression alone.

Take good notes

Many interviewers find this difficult. Some find that it breaks the rapport with the candidates. Later, they find that their memory lets them down, and their recollections are coloured by what they want to believe the candidates said. Others record their own judgements, rather than the facts and statements.

Nevertheless, note down as much as you can. The notes might look something like this:

. . .experiences in psychiatric unit – 2 years – rotation through all sections – frequently took charge – relief in acute area occasionally – had difficulties in persuading psychiatrists to accept new procedures – achieved partial success – operated good rehabilitative practices – limited support from nurse manager – different ideas on care – practically no involvement with learners – prefers research to teaching. . .

Or you may need to record the candidate's verbatim answers to questions (yours or other people's):

Highlight of experience?
   Opening the new unit.
Her contribution?
   Introducing new care plan system.
Main difficulties?
   Selling the idea to charge nurses.
How were they overcome?
   I demonstrated the benefits by setting up a pilot, which they evaluated themselves. (Later admitted that: *It was all set up before I arrived.*)

Sort information under headings

It is useful to set up a matrix as shown in the following example. This example is based on the information gained in the previous section. The criterion column contains all of the criteria that have been set, and the evidence column is intended to give a summary of all of the information that might be used as evidence of whether the criterion is met. We will examine the rating we might give in the next section.

Example

Criterion	Evidence	Rating
Ability to manage change effectively	Experience in persuading psychiatrists to accept new procedures – partially successful only.	
	Implemented new unit care plans, but did not initiate. Says this went well – involved charge nurses and gained their commitment.	
	Oriented to new ideas.	
	Says she is very 'change oriented' and likes to be innovative.	

Beware of over-complicated assessment forms where lots of figures (or ratings) need to be inserted. They rarely work in practice, and are never as scientific as they might look. You do need to have something, though.

Spot the real evidence

Assuming that you know what you are looking for, is all of the information you collect equally useful as a measure of the person's suitability? You need to know what to take seriously, and what to ignore. You need to extricate your own biases and prejudices from the facts. The interview gives both sides scope for generating information that is unreliable as evidence. For instance, the last item in the preceding example – a positive self-rating on a totally predictable requirement – is unreliable. What about the others?

From what the person has done, we can see some evidence that she has been involved in achieving change. We may not be sure how successful this was, because we have to rely on what she says. Probing has revealed that it was not all of her own work. Perhaps the reference, or questioning of the referee, might provide firmer evidence. It is always at this stage that the interviewer realises the questions that should have been asked.

The following example shows a way of rating the quality and kind of evidence obtained.

Example

1 Quality of evidence:

Good evidence

▲ Clearly a proven fact, concrete results quoted.
Apparently a fact, and certainly verifiable.
Many concrete examples quoted.
Despite many opportunities to do so, could not convince us.
One concrete example.
Failed to come up with what was required.
Very much an impression we had.
No evidence to the contrary.
Inferred from something else – we did not really ask.
Reliance on the candidate's word alone.
Evidence both ways.
Not mentioned.
▼ A hunch or speculation on our part – gut feeling.

Poor evidence

2 Direction of evidence:

Evidence of positive (that is, what is required)

▲ Matches criterion.

▼ Does not match criterion.

Evidence of negative (that is, what is not required)

Evidence strategy

You will not be able to secure the highest quality evidence on everything in a short interview. Make sure, however, that you have some solid evidence on the key issues. This is particularly important where you are relying on the interview as your only source of information, to get the strongest evidence you can.

It will be dangerous to make ratings where you have no evidence. Gut feelings are impossible to eradicate. Some people would claim that they are valuable – it is a pity then that they are hardly ever checked out in practice, because the person who gives the 'bad vibes' is always rejected. So, rather than simply seek

211

confirmation, test any gut reaction by seeking evidence to the contrary, before you accept it with your more objective evidence.

The following example illustrates a wide range of quality of evidence (good, reasonable, poor) for the criterion stated.

Example

Criterion	Evidence	Comments
1 Persistence	She said that she was known for never being one to give up.	Poor, unless she can quote some examples to back it up.
2 Persistence	She gave three examples of situations where she insisted that a programme was completed, despite reluctance of some colleagues.	Probably reasonable evidence, if she is truthful – you may check this through the referee.
3 Computer aptitude	Although she had no direct work experience, she was very 'pro' computers, and had bought one for her son.	Poor evidence on aptitude – it might only show a willingness to learn.
4 Computer aptitude	She said she had done the Open University course on computing and achieved very good marks.	If the skills are what is required, and she is truthful, it is good evidence.
5 Ability to listen	She was asked a lot of questions about her approach to patients, but never once mentioned the importance of being a good listener.	Is this a fair test? If you feel that she certainly ought to have mentioned it, then it might be acceptable as reasonable evidence, but you could be wrong to infer too much from this. Often, the things people do unconsciously, they omit to mention.

6	Ability to listen	When asked 'Are you a good listener', she said 'I must be or I wouldn't have got where I am!'	Poor evidence from this leading question, unless she can justify what she means with some detailed concrete examples.
7	Ability to listen	She looked as if she was the kind of person that could be trusted completely with confidences.	Poor evidence. Very much a speculation or gut feeling.
8	Clinical competence	She said she had received the highest scores on all of her assessments to date.	If true (and you can check), it is good evidence, if the standard is the one you require.
9	Planning skills	She had once had to commission a ward, which she did successfully, but if she were to do it again, she would go about it differently.	Probably reasonable evidence.

COMMON ERRORS OF JUDGEMENT

Before we move on to the judgement itself, it will be useful to look at common errors of judgement. The following example gives a summary of the faults that interviewers are prone to, when making judgements, and how they may be remedied. It is based on research findings.

Example

Fault	Remedy
1 No clear selection criteria.	Be clear what you are looking for. Make sure that the signals are valid predictors.
2 The approach is: 'the higher the qualification the better'.	Your standards should describe a range. You should be seeking optimal, not maximal, qualifications.

3	Unsystematic pursuit of evidence.	Plan and structure your interview – probe deeply. Make sure that you are getting the right kind of evidence.
4	People are judged too early, and this is allowed to affect later judgements.	Resist early judgements. Make notes and review them objectively after the interview.
5	People judged positively (or negatively) on one criterion tend to be judged highy (or lowly) on others, irrespective of the evidence – the 'halo' (or 'horns') effect.	Be conscious of this and keep judgements separate from each other.
6	If a good candidate follows a poor one, then judgements are too much affected by the contrast between them – the 'contrast' effect.	Rate everyone on an agreed scale of criteria before comparing them.
7	Interviewers come to different conclusions on the same evidence. Some rate too high, while others rate too low.	Discuss your standards and interpretations with each other and refine them.
8	The opinions of important people affect others' judgements.	Encourage independent ratings and open discussion.
9	Stereotype judgements; for example, people who wear glasses tend to be seen as 'more intelligent', while people who smile a lot are judged more socially skilful.	Resist the tendency – seek a wide range of views. Do not allow yourself to say 'She's a typical ...' or 'So much like so and so'.
10	Some interviewers are much better at judging people 'like us' – that is, of the same sex, age, class and ethnic background. With those who are different, there is a	Generally, distrust 'gut reactions'. Beware of inferring things 'beyond the evidence'.

	tendency to rely on stereotypes and generalisations.	
11	The interview is a fault-finding device. Too much is made of the faults that the interviewers think they've found, thereby ignoring positive qualities.	Seek positive things, as well as negative.
12	Often what people say they do is not what they actually would do.	Use other evidence.

JUDGING AND EVALUATING

The interview is acceptable and open-ended, but it lacks precision as a selection method. A psychologist would say that it is not at all reliable – meaning that it does not produce consistent results. Your ratings will differ from someone else's, even of the same interview. Being open-ended is a mixed blessing. Some of your interview judgements may be no better than if you had tossed a coin.

Psychologists insist on knowing whether we are measuring what we think we are measuring. They call this validity. We are interested in predictive validity, because we are judging future performance. Our ratings are to be seen as signals of future success. We must know that the signals we use are reliable, and that they are good predictors.

Bearing in mind the points made earlier, here is a procedure that can be used for making your judgements.

1 Each panel member sorts out the information she has obtained on each candidate, under the criteria headings. There should be no comment or discussion at this stage.
2 The quality of the evidence in each box is assessed, and if it is acceptable evidence, a rating can be written down, on the lines of:

1 Definitely meets the criterion.
2 Just meets the criterion.
3 Just fails to meet the criterion.
4 Definitely fails to meet the criterion.

215

Interviewers may also want to indicate whether the evidence is overwhelming or scanty. They may sometimes want to say 'No rating because insufficient evidence'. This should not be confused with failure to meet the criterion. Occasionally, a candidate provides no evidence of what is required, despite repeated promptings, or opportunities to do so. In such cases, it is necessary to decide whether this negative evidence means that the criterion has or has not been met.

There may also be contradictory evidence. Some things might point in one direction, others in another. If this is the case, it might be necessary to make a provisional judgement and signal the issues for discussion later.

3 Any issues that need to be discussed further are identified, before making a rating.

4 Taking each candidate at a time, each interviewer systematically lists her scores or ratings on each criterion.

5 Once this has been done, any discrepancies in ratings are identified, and people say why they have made the judgements they have, by quoting their evidence.

6 Discussion then takes place with a view to finding consensus, where there is uncertainty or disagreement. It should not be necessary to discuss the case further when all parties are in close agreement. It is important that this discussion is an open one. The person chairing it must ask open questions in order to explore all of the issues and give everyone the chance to participate.

7 The overall ratings are recorded – with the evidence. The panel may be asked to justify its decision later, and may well be involved in giving feedback to candidates (see Chapter 25).

8 Decisions must then be made on who is 'in the running' or 'above the line'; that is, who meets the criteria set. The reasons for rejection must be stated and recorded. The assessor may then say 'A' or 'B' are acceptable, 'C' and 'D', not. Whether A or B is preferred, depends on the particular requirements.

9 Finally, the panel decides which of the acceptable candidates could be offered the job, and which is the preferred first choice. Here, it may well be that previously minor distinctions come to the fore. It will be certainly necessary to reflect on any particular qualities the candidates can bring, and it

may be decided on fairly marginal issues, such as removal difficulties, the time required for each candidate to become fully effective, or how long the person is likely to stay. Sometimes a very subjective element is introduced here, like 'The person whom I would rather work with', 'This person will fit in better here', or 'The staff will love Y, she's super!'. This may be veiled prejudice, or it may merely reflect the fact that the panel is looking for people like those already there, which could be unwise. Personally, I have a lot more time for people who look at their teams and decide who best complements the current strengths and weaknesses. R M Belbin has emphasised the need to select teams rather than individuals. However, if, after a thorough job of assessment, the panel still feels that there is someone that would prove difficult working with, I would not want to dispute their judgement.

MAKING THE OFFER

If references have not been received and checked, it will be necessary to do this before any offers are made. Perhaps you will want to make contact with the referee quickly by telephone and confirm any things that may still be in doubt.

Although you will want to make the offer as quickly as possible, there is usually no harm in delaying the actual offer by a day or so, if you need to. You might ask whether the candidate has other posts she is considering, and whether she could let you have an answer by a specified time. I would allow the person 24 hours to think about it – she may ask for more. You will not, of course, have turned other acceptable candidates down in the meantime.

Your strategy for negotiating terms with the successful candidate will need to be clear. Take advice from your personnel officer on salary and conditions that can be offered.

Figure 24.1 summarises the steps involved in coming to a decision.

REFERENCE

Belbin, R M, *Management Teams: Why They Succeed or Fail* (Heinemann, 1981).

FURTHER READING

Arvey, Richard D and Campion, James, E 'The employment interview: a summary and review of recent research', *Personnel Psychology*, **35**, 1982.

Bayne, R, 'Can selection interviewing be improved?', *Journal of Occupational Psychology*, **50**(3), 1977.

Carlson, R E, *et al.*, 'Improvements in the selection interview', *Personnel Journal*, **50**(4), 1971.

Curran, M, *Stereotypes and Selection: Gender and Family in the Recruitment Process* (Report for the EOC, 1985).

Morgan, Terry, 'Recent insights into the selection interview', *Personnel Review*, **1**, 1973.

Reading, T, 'How interviews fail', *Management Today*, April 1977.

Shaw, E A, 'Commonality of applicant stereotypes among recruiters', *Personnel Psychology*, **25**(3), 1972.

Schmitt, N, 'Social and situational determinants of interview decisions: implications for the employment interview', *Personnel Psychology*, **29**, 1976.

Ulrich, L and Trumbo, D, 'The selection interview since 1949', *Psychological Bulletin*, **63**, 1965.

Wagner, R F, 'The employment interview, a critical summary', *Personnel Psychology*, **2**, 1949.

Wright, O R, Jnr, 'Summary of research on the selection interview since 1964', *Personal Psychology*, **22**(4), 1969.

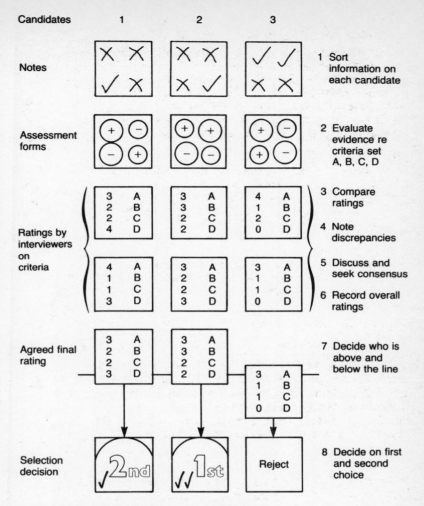

Figure 24.1   *Decision-making summary chart*

Chapter 25

AFTER THE INTERVIEW

Where no counsel is, the people fall: but in the multitude of counsellors there is safety. *Proverbs*

DECIDING TO GIVE FEEDBACK

Interviewers have to make a decision on what to tell unsuccessful candidates after the interview. At the very least, the decision to accept or reject has to be communicated. This can be done in a formal way, by standard letter, which might say 'On this occasion your application has been unsuccessful'. What this might also say to the candidate is 'Don't ask why!'.

Crucial considerations in deciding whether or not to give positive feedback are: whether the candidates want it, and whether the interviewers are willing and capable of responding to the needs of the candidates. A general open-ended commitment to meet people's needs will mean that you are implicitly undertaking to deal with a wide range of needs. Yet failure to give any kind of useful feedback may have consequences.

Many candidates might feel sold short. They may have put a lot of effort into the interview, and perhaps travelled hundreds of miles to be there. They may well feel that to get nothing in return, except perhaps a feeling of resentment and failure, is bad value. They will be disinclined to apply again.

The offer of feedback, on the other hand, signals a caring and well-organised employer:

Well, I didn't get that job, but I liked the way they do things, and if they advertise again, I'll try again.

Thus, there are two areas to be clear about to begin with:

1 What your candidate might want from you.
2 What information or advice you can give.

WHAT INDIVIDUALS MIGHT WANT

We can identify some categories of applicant.

The unsuccessful internal applicant

An internal applicant has even more at stake than someone from outside. Imagine that one of several F-grade sisters applies for one G-grade job in an organisation where there is little opportunity for promotion. Perhaps she has tried for promotion in the past and feels she has been passed over, but is determined to try anyway. Perhaps she believes that the job is hers and that the interview is only a formality. What happens if she does not get the job? Where does she go from here? What if she has to carry on, embarrassed at loss of face in a junior capacity to someone new, maybe even junior to a job she has been doing her best at for months previously. This is a problem of readjustment, which requires skilled counselling. In most cases, the sister's manager will have a key role to play.

The unconfident job hunter

A mature person returning to nursing after a break will probably be competing with individuals who have learnt to put themselves across confidently. Here, the requirement might focus on the individual's presentation of herself at the interview: how she handled the questions, whether she gave appropriate and convincing answers – whether, in fact, she has made the best of herself.

The inexperienced, aspiring nurse

She will be applying for promotion. She will want to know whether she was in the running to begin with. Having got herself shortlisted, did she fail to come across well in person, and if so, why? What were the ratings she received? Was she appointable, but pipped at the post by someone marginally better – or was she far short of the requirements? If the latter is

221

the case, she needs to know what to do about it. Was it the wrong kind of post, or was she simply not ready?

The square peg

Some individuals fail chronically to establish their credibility at the interview. No one wants to tell them why. It may be prejudice on the part of the panel, or simply that the person is unable to create the necessary confidence in her abilities. Characteristically, such people produce an outstanding application, and there is a feeling of disappointment when they do not live up to it in person. Each failure rubs more salt into the wound. The person becomes prickly and easily hurt – she develops a mission on the lines of 'I'm in a hurry to get on! Why doesn't someone tell me what they don't like about me? Where am I going wrong?'

Irrespective of the type of candidate, some factors always apply.

Encouragement

Once rejected, some candidates might conclude that they are unacceptable. This may be far from the case – you may, in fact, want them to apply again. If this is the case, you will want the opportunity to set the record straight, to encourage them to reapply for a more suitable job, or when they are ready. The conversation you have will be helpful to both parties.

Principles

As a service that espouses caring principles, it is appropriate to respect an individual's right to know how she is being seen and judged, and to support her growth.

Supportiveness

It is in nobody's interests for candidates not only to fail to do justice to themselves, but to lose confidence in the process.

Feedback to the interviewer

As an interviewer, it should be important to you to find out how you came across to candidates, and also whether your judgements might have been made too hastily. It is a good discipline to be able to justify your decision to the candidate. The rigour and clarity that this process implies will go some way to ensuring that your decisions are fully defensible – for example at industrial tribunals. In other words, your feedback to the candidate has to be good, and based on proper evidence. Clearly, this should tighten up your evaluation of candidates and lead you to better selection decisions. Incidentally, there will also be a need to ensure that panellists agree in their detailed judgements.

FEEDBACK, ADVICE OR COUNSELLING?

It is important that you make it clear to begin with what you are offering to candidates. This is encapsulated in the first offer made; for instance:

If you would like to know how you came across to us, we will let you know.

If there is anything you want to talk to us about afterwards, please feel free to do so.

Mr X, the assessor, is offering advice to any candidates who might find it helpful.

Note that in the last case the word 'offer' is used, rather than 'give' feedback or advice.

What you say at the outset is very important. You must create the context. Perhaps the term 'advice' is best, since it may not in fact involve counselling.

DIFFERING AIMS IN POST-INTERVIEW COUNSELLING

Whoever is to offer the advice or counselling, the panel should agree on what they are offering each candidate:

- The applicant may be offered support in getting over some of the feelings that may have come to the fore.
- She may be offered a clear idea of where the panel thinks she scored or did not.
- She may receive advice on how she might progress in her career.

What is offered will differ from one candidate to the next. Internal candidates will probably need – and may even demand

223

– a much more elaborate counselling session than external candidates. Many candidates will opt out of the opportunity altogether. Lastly, but more importantly, the interviewers will learn the applicant's views of the interview – and this you should welcome.

It might be helpful to structure the process into four possible levels:

1 Level one involves advising the person on how she came over, which is offering information about what the person said and did, and how it was perceived. There is no need to go beyond this unless both parties choose to.
2 Level two involves sharing the actual judgements made about the candidate, in particular whether the person was 'above the line' or not. It is an open response to 'Why I didn't get the job'.
3 Level three is concerned with being able to share and help release hurt or angry feelings, which may be aimed at the panel or self.
4 Level four offers help for the future – either in making a better presentation or re-evaluating the person's career objectives.

Dealing with raw feelings

For many candidates, the process is disturbing and unsettling. The aftermath can involve feelings of disappointment, loss or anger. As an interviewer, you may not feel able to deal with these feelings. You may feel that you are not in a position to deal with the anger and insecurities of people that you have met briefly, and made quick judgements about at the interview. You may not think it appropriate for the executioner to be the one to comfort the victim.

You may thus fear getting drawn into a counselling situation with a stranger. You may fear arguments where you have to justify a judgement that is hotly denied by the candidate. 'No, you got me all wrong, I'm not like that at all.' You may find it hard to avoid being drawn into comparisons with other candidates. 'Surely I had more experience to offer than so and so.' As an interviewer, you will want to make sure that there are some boundaries. The skilled counsellor almost intuitively knows how to avoid being drawn into offering advice to people whom she will not be able to help. She picks up cues that inform her of what approach to take.

What does the skilled adviser do?

Here is a cameo example of one approach at levels one and two:

Thank you for ringing me. Do you want to talk about the interview? How do you think it went? Really, why do you think that? That's interesting, that isn't quite how you came across to us. Why do I say that? Well, for instance, you said (and I noted this) that you found it hard. . . . You seemed anxious when we talked about. . . . Yes, perhaps we read too much into those remarks, and I accept that it wasn't quite what you meant to say, but that was the impression we got from you. No, we didn't think you were quite ready for this post. You'll understand that I'm not in a position to reveal the precise discussion the panel had, but that was our conclusion.

Levels three and four are primarily concerned with good listening, but the adviser might be heard to say things like:

You showed us a lot of strengths, such as. . . . What makes you think that? Well, I think I can understand how you feel. It must be disappointing after the effort you have put in. Might I suggest that it might be possible to look at what happened in a different light. Are you really sure it is what you want? I sense that I am not getting across to you at the moment, would you like to talk more about this tomorrow?

It is beyond the scope of this book to identify an overall approach to personal or career counselling in detail. I think it must be seen as a joint problem-solving exercise, with the whole context of the candidate's application and the candidate's feelings about the outcome of the interview as concrete starting points. The following checklist gives six essentials for post-interview counselling. You will find further advice in the references at the end of this chapter.

Checklist 25.1

1 Timing:
There are two issues here. One is that, ideally, there needs to be a little space for the candidate to settle and reflect between interview and counselling. On the other hand, you may prefer to talk to the individual after the interview in person, rather than on the telephone the next day. (I can think of some, however, for whom the opposite might be true!) You also need enough time to be able to listen.

2　Sensitivity:
This means giving attention to the applicant's feelings, and not being put off by anger or bitterness, which may need to come out before there can be any moving ahead. Whether the feelings are simply the background to your discussion on the interviewee's performance, or have to be worked through fully during a deeper counselling session, will depend on the level at which you want to work. Each interviewer will decide whether she feels it appropriate to take on the latter. Often, it will not be.

3　Openness:
This means that the adviser is prepared to take criticism from the applicant: 'The questions were not clear to me'; 'You didn't seem really interested in what I said.' Also, that when necessary, the adviser can be frank with the candidate: 'You may think that's what you said, but it isn't what we heard.'

4　Positiveness:
This means concentrating on what was well done, highlighting strengths: 'You warmed up at once when you were telling us about rehabilitating that lady who had had a stroke.'

5　Fairness:
This means balancing and confronting issues that are awkward.

6　Specificity:
This means giving clear and detailed feedback. It could also mean providing detailed advice on future career progress. Always have concrete examples ready to quote when you want to reflect back on something to the candidate. This involves saying 'You said that...' rather than 'You seemed...'. Your judgements should pertain to evidence rather than impression.

At this stage, you might find it useful to look again at the examples of imaginary dialogue given earlier to check which of these principles are involved.

PRACTICAL ISSUES

Who offers the feedback?

If there is an external assessor, it is usual for this person to do this. Where the interview panel is made up of local managers, then it is generally the most senior person who will offer to see the applicants.

The choice must be sensitive to the individuals concerned, and not one that generates any suspicion or anxiety on the part of any candidate. Sometimes there will be good reasons for choosing someone other than the assessor or most senior person. The content of what is said by someone on behalf of a panel should be agreed by the panel.

When and where should it take place?

Create the best opportunity you can. It may have to be a five-minute telephone call to the other end of the country, but it could sometimes be a useful session in a quiet room away from the office, when you are not too busy.

The problem of relationships

Do you know the candidate? Perhaps you have a working relationship already:

Whenever I appear on the ward, Sister Brown disappears. Everyone knows that we don't really get on. My nerve fails me at the thought of sitting down with her and discussing why she didn't get the job. She's just not up to it and she can't see why.

The nettle must be grasped, and if you are the person to do it, you will not be able to shirk it. In the foregoing case, there is a tension that is likely to be damaging until the issues are allowed into the open. You do need to think carefully in such situations about the approach you use, and be very aware of the feelings – anger, loss of face, distrust or embarrassment – you might have to deal with.

Who is competent?

Most interviewers have some anxieties:

I'm not really sure how to go about it. What if we have a maverick applicant who 'sets up' the panel? What if we have an angry applicant who doesn't like the way she's been interviewed, and thinks that she never stood a chance anyway with an all-female panel?

What if I am asked about the other candidates?

What if she denies our judgement or argues the decision?

Will I have to reveal our disagreements?

How can I be positive – she was simply awful.

227

Again, the tough issues may not be shirked. If the adviser believes this was a maverick applicant who had not prepared or thought about the job and was wasting everyone's time, she must have the courage to say so.

If you are clear about what you are doing, and pick up cues from the candidate, you are likely to stay within your depth, and this is important. You will want to be as frank and open as you can, but you may also need sticking points – if you cannot tell the candidate what she wants to know, say so.

Most applicants will be genuine and will want to come away with a sense of self-respect. In the main, they will be keen to learn from experience and, like you, will want to end on a constructive note.

The personality that is hard to relate to

The angry person will often not be listening – the conversation may be unfruitful, but it is likely to be brief. 'I'm sorry, but that is the conclusion we came to' might be the closing remark.

It may, in fact, be much harder to help an applicant of gentle and apparently unassertive nature, or someone who earnestly seeks promotion, but lacks the energy and leadership quality that the job needs. The person who believes that long and loyal service justifies promotion is known to many organisations. You can only try to find the best ways to use her skills.

Evidence and snap judgements

The quality of the evidence you have available is crucial, of course, if you are to do a good job. Very unflattering comments are often made after interviews.

He'd be all right for some places, but he'd never fit in here.

She's as mad as a hatter!

I wouldn't put her in charge of a wagon load of monkeys!

She'd go at things like a bull at a gate!

Did you hear that outright lie?

In spite of 'gut reactions', you will need to separate evidence from mere opinion.

You will have a set of detailed notes on what each candidate said and did, to refer to. These are invaluable in any feedback session.

You will be relating responses to your criteria in order to judge who could do the job. You will appreciate applicant A's personal charm, but recognise that she did not actually answer the questions. You will try to judge whether applicant B's tense manner was due to interview nerves or is an inherent part of her character. Would it put off the consultants? She clearly knows what the job entails.

You will test out each others' opinions, check your scoring, agree your decision and check references. If you have done this process thoroughly, then you will have a verdict that can be well supported from the evidence. The candidate, too, will usually then tend to see your verdict as objective, even if unpalatable. It will probably not be a surprise.

In this way, the very fact of having to give feedback may sharpen the panel's judgements in the future. Interviews are rich sources of learning for both parties. The same attitudes of respect and care that nurses apply to patients should apply to staff just as much.

Figure 25.1 summarises the issues that need to be considered in post-interview feedback.

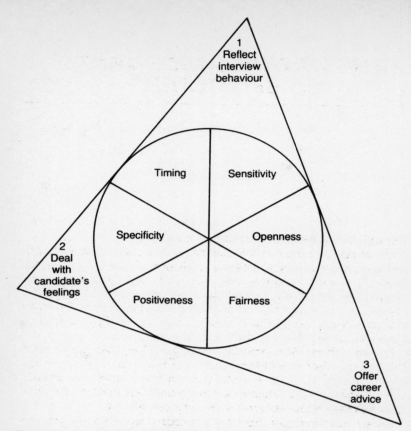

Figure 25.1 *Post-interview feedback summary chart*

THE DAY OF JUDGEMENT –
EPILOGUE

The story of Sally Robinson, candidate, continued.

A year later, Sally got exactly the job she wanted. By that time, she had gained confidence at interviews, although it took several more failures before she really managed to do so. She now has a clear idea of what they are all about, she knows how she can best put herself across, she prepares well, and she gets there in plenty of time. 'They are a challenge, but they do not scare me any longer,' she says, 'I know what I have to do and say.'

On the occasion that she was successful, Sally was surprised to find Shirley Garnett interviewing her again. This time, however, Shirley was no longer hesitant and unprepared – she was firmly in control, asked good questions, and made Sally feel at ease. But then, Sally was that much easier to interview the second time.

Shirley had moved on from her previous post. It was her experience as a candidate for her new post that made her think a lot about what was really involved in interviewing. When, recently, she had to select her new team, she studied everything she could find about recruitment and selection. She went on courses, looked at herself on video and got people who were better than her to give her comments on her style. Now she has picked the people, she is quietly checking whether the predictions she made about each of them were correct. She has kept her rating sheets and records of interviews for this purpose.

Miss Williams has not done anything to change her interviewing ideas, or her ideas on anything else, for that matter. However, she has made one major change in her life – she has retired from the service.

CRITERIA-BASED INTERVIEW ASSESSMENT FORM

Name of candidate: *Post*:

Criteria ::		*Assessment* ::::::::::::::::::::::::::::::::::	
Requirement	Details and standards	Evidence found	Rating
1			
2			
3			
4			
5			
6			

Note

You can specify criteria using the CCR method (Chapter 16) to define:

- Competency requirements: What the person must be *able* to do.
- Commitment requirements: interests, compatibility, confidence, application, circumstances; that is, what the person must be *willing to do*.

Alternatively, you can use the seven-point plan categories, or invent your own.

NURSING COMPETENCIES

The Nurses, Midwives and Health Visitors Rules Approval Order 1983: Extract from Statutory Instrument 1983 No. 873: Training for admission to Parts 1 to 8 of the register.

18　1　Courses leading to a qualification the successful completion of which shall enable an application to be made for admission to Part 1, 3, 5 or 8 of the register shall provide opportunities to enable the student to accept responsibility for her personal professional development and to acquire the competencies required to:

a　advise on the promotion of health and the prevention of illness;

b　recognise situations that may be detrimental to the health and well-being of the individual;

c　carry out those activities involved when conducting the comprehensive assessment of a person's nursing requirements;

d　recognise the significance of the observations made and use these to develop an initial nursing assessment;

e　devise a plan of nursing care based on the assessment with the co-operation of the patient, to the extent that this is possible, taking into account the medical prescription;

f　implement the planned programme of nursing care and where appropriate teach and co-ordinate other members of the caring team who may be responsible for implementing specific aspects of the nursing care;

g　review the effectiveness of the nursing care provided, and where appropriate, initiate any action that may be required;

h　work in a team with other nurses, and with medical and para-medical staff and social workers;

i   undertake the management of the care of a group of patients over a period of time and organise the appropriate support services

related to the care of the particular type of patient with whom she is likely to come in contact when registered in that Part of the register for which the student intends to qualify.

18 2 Courses leading to a qualification the successful completion of which shall enable an application to be made for admission to Part 2, 4, 6 or 7 of the register shall be designed to prepare the student to undertake nursing care under the direction of a person registered in Part 1, 3, 5 or 8 of the register and provide opportunities for the student to develop the competencies required to:

a   assist in carrying out comprehensive observation of the patient and help in assessing her care requirements;
b   develop skill to enable her to assist in the implementation of nursing care under the direction of a person registered in Part 1, 3, 5 or 8 of the register;
c   accept delegated nursing tasks;
d   assist in reviewing the effectiveness of the care provided;
e   work in a team with other nurses, and with medical and para-medical staff and social workers

related to the care of the particular type of patient with whom she is likely to come into contact when registered in that Part of the register for which the student intends to qualify.

LIST OF USEFUL ADDRESSES

English National Board for
Nursing, Midwifery and Health
Visiting
Victory House
170 Tottenham Court Road
London W1P 0HA
071 388 3131

National Board for Nursing,
Midwifery and Health
Visiting for Northern Ireland
79 Chichester Street
Belfast BT1 4JE
0232 238152

National Board for Nursing,
Midwifery and Health
Visiting for Scotland
22 Queen Street
Edinburgh EH2 1JX
031 226 7371

United Kingdom Central Council
for Nursing, Midwifery and
Health Visiting
23 Portland Place
London W1A 1BA
071 637 7181

Welsh National Board for
Nursing, Midwifery and Health
Visiting
Floor 13
Pearl Assurance House
Greyfriars Road
Cardiff CF1 3AG
0222 395535

Continuing Nurse Education
Programme
26 Danbury Street
London N1 8JU
071 354 3718

English National Board Careers
Advisory Centre
PO Box 356
Sheffield S8 0SJ
0742 551064

Institute of Personnel Management
35 Camp Road
London SW19 4UX
081 946 9100

Commission for Racial Equality
Elliot House
10–12 Allington Street
London SW1E 5EH
071 828 7022

Equal Opportunities Commission
Overseas House
Quay Street
Manchester M3 3NM
061 833 9244

Nursing Times
4 Little Essex Street
London WC2R 3LF
071 240 1101 (advertising)
071 379 0970 (editorial)
0256 29242 (subscriptions)

Health and Social Services Journal
4 Little Essex Street
London WC2R 3LF
071 836 6633
0256 29242 (subscriptions)

INDEX TO CHECKLISTS AND SUMMARY CHARTS

INDEX

241